Hyperhidrosis

A Comprehensive Guide to Diagnosis and Treatment

(Safe Ways to Stop Excessive Sweating Excessive Sweating Causes)

Juan Humble

I0089844

Published By **Oliver Leish**

Juan Humble

Hyperhidrosis: A Comprehensive Guide to Diagnosis and Treatment (Safe Ways to Stop Excessive Sweating Excessive Sweating Causes)

ISBN 978-1-7782476-7-5

Legal & Disclaimer

The information contained in this book is not designed to replace or take the place of any form of medicine or professional medical advice. The information in this book has been provided for educational & entertainment purposes only.

The information contained in this book has been compiled from sources deemed reliable, and it is accurate to the best of the Author's knowledge; however, the Author cannot guarantee its accuracy and validity and cannot be held liable for any errors or omissions. Changes are periodically made to this book. You must consult your doctor or get professional medical advice before using any of the suggested remedies, techniques, or information in this book.

Table Of Contents

Chapter 1: Understanding Sweat

Before you could in truth recognize how hyperhidrosis rise up and a manner to deal with it, you want to apprehend perspiration and the manner it really works.

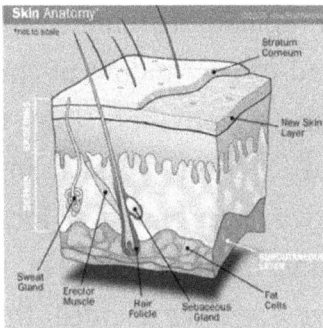

Perspiration is the production of the human frame of fluid that is more frequently than not composed of water (further to numerous dissolved solids) which are excreted through way of the sweat glands. There are averagely 2 to 4 million sweat glands which may be allotted all through your frame. The majority of these sweat glands are called eccrine glands which might be placed in large numbers within the soles of the ft, the hands, the cheeks, the forehead, and inside the armpits.

These eccrine glands will secrete a clean and odourless fluid it's sweat. Sweating will permit your body to regulate its middle temperature. It is controlled in the middle of the preoptic and anterior regions of the thoughts's hypothalamus. This is in which thermosensitive neurons are located. Our nerves will ship signs to motive the sweat glands to provide sweat once they collect stimuli like:

• Message from thoughts that it's miles too warm

• Hormones

• Emotions

• Physical hobby or workout

The unique shape of sweat glands is apocrine glands. These are specially determined in the armpits and the genital regions. They normally produce thick fluid that once it comes in contact with bacteria, it's going to in all likelihood produce a characteristic body smell.

Sweat consists not specially of water, but with exceptional minerals or compounds. It can also incorporate lactate and urea. Mineral composition will variety with each individual. This is predicated upon at the acclimation to warmth, workout, the perfect strain supply, the length of sweating, and the composition of the minerals in the frame.

For people who have immoderate perspiration trap 22 scenario or hyperhidrosis, the sweat glands (particularly the eccrine glands) will overreact to the stimuli. With this, they have a tendency to grow to be overactive and produce more sweat than ordinary or vital. Usually, individuals who be troubled by using hyperhidrosis are defined to be "usually on" in phrases in their perspiration production.

HYPERHIDROSIS DEFINED

Hyperhidrosis is a systematic situation wherein it's far characterised by using excessive sweating. The frame will produce some distance more sweat that what is needed or required to modify the temperature of the frame.

Sweat glands are discovered within the skin all over the frame, however there are better numbers of these glands in areas of the body much like the arms, ft, armpits, and genital area. Perspiration or sweating is a normal response of the body for temperature law. It is managed through the worried device as a physiologic response on the identical time as the inner of body temperature rises. Exposure to excessive environmental temperature or workout will frequently cause perspiration. In situations whilst you're exceedingly harassed, sweat glands also are because of manner of the anxious tool to supply sweat, specially inside the arms and ft. It is everyday for human beings to excessively sweat whilst nerve-racking or has a fever. Yet, those physiologic responses do not purpose excessive sweating. However, in hyperhidrosis sufferers, the stimulation of the sweat glands to offer sweat is hyperactive.

Usually, this condition begins in youngsters or the early years of children. The scenario then will become extra severe or immoderate with puberty and into adulthood. Men and ladies can likely experience this scientific situation. Reports said that 1% of adults have hyperhidrosis. The signs and symptoms and signs and symptoms of hyperhidrosis will appear at some point of adolescence and stay moderate or development in severity for the duration of maturity. It is uncommon that symptoms and symptoms and signs and symptoms will appear suddenly in maturity.

Apart from hyperhidrosis, immoderate sweating can signal that someone has thyroid hassle, low blood sugar, and unique annoying device problems.

CATEGORIES

enerally, Hyperhidrosis is classed into two classes- Primary Focal and Secondary Generalized. Learning about those training will assist you recognize more how this scientific scenario takes place. The distinction the various two categories should be nicely understood to understand the pathology of the kind of medical scenario.

Primary Focal Hyperhidrosis

Primary focal hyperhidrosis is noted immoderate sweating that isn't because of every different underlying scientific condition nor a issue or negative impact of any pharmacologic agent. This definitely technique that that the excessive sweating is the medical circumstance itself. The type sweating that takes place is generally on specific regions termed as "focal regions." Symmetric occurrence enormously takes location due to this that the left and right elements of the frame is affected in addition. The commonplace focal regions are the fingers, toes, underarms, face, and head.

This class of hyperhidrosis generally starts offevolved to arise in some unspecified time in the future of young people or teens, usually in the focal areas of the toes and palms. It is thrilling to phrase that at the equal time as human beings with number one focal hyperhidrosis will revel in excessive sweating as a minimum as soon as each week, they don't usually immoderate sweating in some unspecified time in the future of sleep. Primary focal hyperhidrosis is likewise inherited to family people. The hereditary detail of this beauty of hyperhidrosis has by no means been conclusive with research as of the instantaneous.

As referred to, the regions which is probably at risk of number one focal hyperhidrosis are the face, underarms, fingers, and ft.

Facial hyperhidrosis. Most typically, facial hyperhidrosis can purpose someone to sweat copiously on the face to the quantity that sweat is dripping regardless of slight exertion. This each impacts males and females.

Sweating additionally arise at the scalp. Contrary to well-known notion facial immoderate sweating first-rate takes area to obese human beings and to human beings after social embarrassment or anxiety, it's miles normally held that facial hyperhidrosis is genetically and now not due to outside reasons.

Embarrassment and uneasiness are commonly the feelings of people with facial hyperhidrosis in order that they keep away from social touch and exposure simply to keep away from sweating. For girls, they typically have brief haircut and avoid putting on make-up. While some bring around towels, others will take frequent showers to revel in easy and be relieved. People with facial hyperhidrosis have immoderate anxiety stages and characteristic low vanity. They are constantly concerned that their apparel or collars in their shirts can be soaked with sweat. They regularly enjoy burning or reddening in their eyes as salty sweat seeps in them.

Axillary hyperhidrosis. Visible underarm sweat earrings are the hassle of humans with axillary hyperhidrosis. This phenomenon of excessive sweating within the underarms is called axillary hyperhidrosis. This is at the identical time as the aggravating device will "over-activate" the sweat glands of the axilla (underarms) ensuing in excessive sweating inside the underarms. People with axillary hyperhidrosis will keep away from the use of precise sorts of clothes, fabrics, or hues.

This usually starts offevolved earlier than someone reaches his or her teen years. At that age, this could sincerely endorse derision and entertainment among friends. The sufferer will revel in emotional pressure that results to being socially inept in some unspecified time within the destiny of maturity and hassle in regarding specific human beings.

Palmar hyperhidrosis. This is the excessive sweating of the palms delivered on once more through the over-activation of the sweat glands. Usually, people with this form of hyperhidrosis avoid shaking palms. They will experience awkward at the same time as protecting a glass bottle, guidance the wheel in their car, or maybe gripping the staircase rail. Daily obligations that involved the use of the arms might be very uncomfortable for them. They will experience embarrassed and harassed in the occasion that they dedicate mistakes because of their sweaty fingers.

Many people professional having sweaty hands due to anxiety or anxiousness. However, humans with palmar hyperhidrosis, they normally hands soaking with sweat always. The onset of this syndrome is usually at some point of youth. It is belief to be hereditary.

Chapter 2: Prevalence & Incidence

The modern epidemiologic records on Hyperhidrosis is scarce and inconclusive. The costs and information in numerous opinions and studies do no longer clear reflect the actual incidence of this medical state of affairs. Precise occurrence or impact estimates stays vague, but there are more studies which may be being completed up top this contemporary.

In america, a mailed survey modified into despatched to 100 fifty,000 households. It modified into projected to the us populace based definitely totally on US census. This survey modified into finished through Dee Anna Glaser, MD., a professor of dermatology in the University of Saint Louis. The survey modified into completed to decide the prevalence of hyperhidrosis and to evaluate the impact of sweating on the ones affected by axillary hyperhidrosis. Although this survey modified into finished a few years in the past, the outcomes will surely show off how not unusual hyperhidrosis is.

All the outcomes accrued had been posted in an hassle of Journal of the American Academy of Dermatology. According to Glaser, there have been an predicted 7.Eight million human beings inside the United States who be afflicted by hyperhidrosis.

There is an expected 2.Eight% of the population in US who've primary focal hyperhidrosis. Hyperhidrosis will typically have an impact on every men and women, specifically within the a long term between 25 to sixty four years vintage. Several also can had been with this medical scenario while you remember that teenagers.

Hyperhidrosis isn't always any connected with mortality. Although, the more excessive and critical times of hyperhidrosis can substantially have an effect on a victim's incredible of life.

RISK FACTORS

Here are the threat factors for hyperhidrosis.

Genetics. Because the etiology of primary focal hyperhidrosis is unknown, it's miles more frequently than no longer related to genetics. Some people inherit the tendency of excessive sweating, in particular at the soles in their ft and arms in their arms. If one you enjoy this scientific situation, it's miles likely that simply one in all your circle of relatives contributors might also moreover have this identical hassle. The problem is even family participants don't talk to every one of a kind approximately they hyperhidrosis dilemma.

Medical Conditions Associated with Sweating	Medical Conditions Associated with Sweating
Infections • HIV • Tuberculosis • Bacterial (eg. endocarditis, abscesses, tubercular disease, osteomyelitis) • Fungal (eg. histoplasmosis, coccidioidomycosis) **Malignancy** • Lymphomas • Miscellaneous cancers **Endocrine disorders** • Hyperthyroidism • Hyperpituitarism • Pheochromocytoma • Carcinoid syndrome • Diabetes insipidus • Hypoglycemia • Acromegaly • Pregnancy • Menopause	**Neurologic disorders** • Stroke • Peripheral (autonomic) neuropathy • Spinal injury • Parkinson's disease **Miscellaneous** • Gustatory sweating • Angina • Respiratory failure • Panic disorder • Esophageal reflux • Drug or alcohol withdrawal • Anxiety disorders • Rheumatologic disease (eg. temporal arteritis, Takayasu's arteritis)

All races can be tormented by hyperhidrosis. However, medical critiques evidenced that Japanese people are 20 instances extra often with hyperhidrosis in evaluation to specific races.

Sex. Both male and ladies are at threat to have hyperhidrosis.

Age. Persons of each age may additionally have hyperhidrosis. However, primary focal hyperhidrosis commonly start all through teens or young adults. There have become a have a study that become performed that located greater of the human beings surveyed stated that they have their excessive sweating trouble considering the reality that earlier than they will recollect. Some said for the reason that puberty and others for the duration of adulthood.

ETIOLOGY

Though, in our lack of knowledge, we often loosely use the term "sweat problem" to the ones folks who are displaying the signs and symptoms and signs and symptoms and signs and symptoms of hyperhidrosis with out understanding that their problem is past only a easy catch 22 situation. They are suffering from this immoderate clinical trouble that requires proper scientific analysis and treatment.

The lack of information approximately the hyperhidrosis sprouted from the dearth of records of what motives this scientific circumstance. So what motives someone to have hyperhidrosis?

Under ordinary situations, the hypothalamus (this is the part of the thoughts that is chargeable for the law of sweat-associated capabilities) sends sensory alerts to the sweat nerves. The sweat nerves (part of the sympathetic nervous device located inside the chest cavity), in flip, will deliver symptoms to the sweat glands causing the latter to offer sweat. Consequently, because of hyperhidrosis, the sweat glands will disobey the indicators because it have been and produce high-quality quantity of amount. Then this excellent quantity of sweat will are seeking stores on areas like your fingers, toes, underarms, or perhaps your trunk region.

In primary hyperhidrosis, there is no real etiology. It is truly attributed to the genetic predisposition of households.

On the opposite hand, secondary hyperhidrosis takes place due to an underlying medical condition or medicinal drugs. The sweating that takes area is both anywhere within the frame or truly confined in a selected vicinity. Some conditions and pharmacologic dealers which might be regularly related with secondary hyperhidrosis are the following:

Neurologic Injuries. Acute spinal harm can cause the lack of sweating below the net web website of harm. However, it is able to also cause localized areas of hyperhidrosis which could take region months or years after the damage. Patients with spinal wire harm at or above T6 may also have autonomic dysreflexia with which they may experience immoderate sweating at the face and the top part of the trunk. Central concerned tool injuries also can reason hyperhidrosis. Strokes can end end result to hemispheric or medullary infarcts important to hyperhidrosis in the ipsilateral and contralateral facets, respectively. On the aother hand, injury to the cranial a part of the sympathetic chain can result in the hyperhidrosis at the face, neck, and shoulder.

Metabolic problems or procedures. Diseases like thyrotoxicosis, diabetes mellitus, hypoglycaemia, gout, pheochromocytoma, and menopause can motive the onset of hyperhidrosis. Women present manner menopause enjoy hot flashes. Some of them also can additionally be wake up within the middle of the night through the use of soaking sweats and chills. Hypoglycemia or low blood sugar can purpose hyperhidrosis. Many diabetics who're depending on insulin or oral anti-diabetic will revel in low blood sugar at night time discovered by means of the use of immoderate sweating. An over energetic thyroid gland can reason excessive sweating as the boom within the metabolic price of the body in flip growth the frame's temperature.

Parkinson's infection. The excessive sweating of man or woman's with Parkinson's illness takes area concurrently with the decrease in the activation of the sweat glands within the fingers of the hand. This will suggest that the axial hyperhidrosis is a compensatory phenomenon for the reduced characteristic inside the extremities.

Hodgkin's sickness. In each degree of Hodgkin's ailment, the person B diploma ought to have normal symptoms and signs and symptoms of the disorder that is commonly fever and night time sweats.

Infections. Infectious illnesses like tuberculosis, systemic fungal infections, osteomyelitis, AIDS, abscesses, and endocarditis can result in secondary generalized hyperhidrosis. Tuberculosis has night time time sweats as considered one of its signs and symptoms, coupled with fever and cough.

Chronic Alcoholism. Alcohol will act as a depressant of the important disturbing gadget. It can motive sweating and can mess up the thermoregulation mechanism of the mind. Excessive sweating typically happens even as alcohol is stopped. Aside from hyperhidrosis, an alcoholic may additionally even revel in nausea, shaking, anxiety, progressed blood strain, hallucinations, and seizures (delirium tremens).

Febrile Illnesses. There are severa motives for fever to get up. But normally, as your frame temperature increase, you frequently sweat notably. This is your frame's compensatory mechanism to get rid of more warm temperature. This is a ordinary reaction of the body. But repeated episodes of fever, chills, and sweating will recommend excessive contamination.

Cancers. Nights sweats can be an early symptom of some types of cancers which incorporates lymphoma and leukemia.

Medications. The use of pharmacologic sellers can affect one or greater additives of the human thermoregulation and this will result in the superiority of hyperhidrosis. Medications which consist of propanolol, physostigmine, pilocarpine, tricyclic antidepressants, and serotonin reuptake inhibitors were counseled to motive excessive sweating. The drug referred to as Efavirenz turned into currently described to bring about nocturnal sweating this is resolved with the aid of tapering the dosage.

WHEN TO SEEK MEDICAL HELP

If you consider you studied which you are experiencing or affected by hyperhidrosis, you need to are looking for clinical hobby or intervention right away.

Chapter 3: Signs & Symptoms

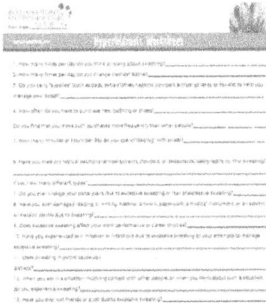

As you can have acknowledged already (due to the previous segment), hyperhidrosis can both continue to be in a constrained place or have an effect on a large part of the body. Areas with large numbers of sweat glands include the axilla, fingers, toes, and the groin region are the most touchy elements that hyperhidrosis can arise.

Main signs and signs and symptoms and symptoms and signs and signs and symptoms of hyperhidrosis will encompass:

•Frequent, observable, excessive perspiration that might soak via clothing.

•Abnormally excessive sweating on your toes, underarms, head and face that can be bothersome.

•Clamminess or dripping of sweat droplets at the fingers of the arms or the soles of the toes.

The immoderate perspiration can in reality disrupt your sports of each day living. The episodes of excessive sweating can typically get up at the least as quickly as each week without any apparent purpose.

Other signs and symptoms and signs and signs and symptoms accompanying excessive perspiration are:

•Skin Maceration. As hyperhidrosis can cause dehydration and pores and skin issues, it is able to result in the maceration of the pores and pores and skin due to contamination ensuing to sturdy odors.

•Fissuring and Scaling. These may be said with profuse sweating. The hands of the fingers and the soles of the toes will typically enjoy cracks, fissures, and scales due to an excessive amount of perspiration.

•Extreme dryness. After episodes of profuse sweating, the skin will commonly dry up.

•Temperature versions. There is a difference of pores and skin temperature wherein immoderate sweating takes place in comparison to exclusive regions of the frame.

With these particular signs and signs and symptoms and signs and symptoms and symptoms, the clinician or your medical scientific doctor can now help in diagnosing your hyperhidrosis situation.

The International Hyperhidrosis Society offers a worksheet (see subsequent page) for hyperhidrosis patients on the way to hold tune or show their excessive perspiration and the way it impairs their daily sports activities. Keeping track of your hyperhidrosis each day consequences will now not super assist you, however may also assist your scientific doctor or clinician in diagnosing. This mode of monitoring can be evidence to your circle of relatives and friends of the way hyperhidrosis negatively influences you. You also can hire this worksheet as proof for your medical medical medical health insurance business company if you need them to devise to cowl your treatments.

DIAGNOSING AND MEDICAL EXAMINATIONS

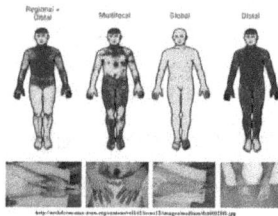

Most patients who are experiencing immoderate sweating or hyperhidrosis will visit a dermatologist, except if she or he is suffering from an underlying medical situation (typically visit a scientific clinical doctor).

Your doctor (or dermatologist) will typically begin with a scientific fitness data and a physical exam. This is the start of the diagnostic device. The medical healthy facts will include a circle of relatives fitness facts. Studies have examined that 25% to 50% sufferers with hyperhidrosis (specially palmar) have a family statistics of the sickness. The scientific health practitioner will ask approximately the location, time patterns, and triggers of your excessive sweating thru the healthful facts taking.

In the physical exam, your health practitioner will probably see sweat droplets to your body even on the identical time as you aren't demanding and feature a normal heart rate. If your signs and signs are very obvious, it's far quite smooth of your doctor to diagnose hyperhidrosis.

Laboratory Tests. Your physician will order blood assessments and different laboratory exams. This is to rule out any immoderate scientific situations that may have cause your excessive sweating.

For very excessive hyperhidrosis, your medical doctor will recommend precise checks to pinpoint the regions in which sweating is originates. These exams are the gravimetric dimension, Minor-starch Iodine take a look at and Thermoregulatory sweat test. They will help the medical medical doctor to advantage facts this is useful in considering and the use of remedy techniques.

Gravimetric Measurement. This is a quantitative technique in measuring the severity of perspiration in a affected man or woman. This may be completed at the palm or the axilla. However, it's miles vital to phrase that this measurement method isn't accomplished as a routine clinical check, however in medical trials handiest.

After drying the region, a pre-weighed filter out paper is finished to the palm or axilla and timed the usage of a stopwatch. The clean out paper is then weighed in order that the fee of sweat manufacturing can be measured in mg/min.

Sweating costs of everyday people and hyperhidrosis patients are provided right here:

Minor-starch Iodine Test. This test entails utilising starch to the pores and pores and skin coupled with iodine. The regions with immoderate sweating will have a propensity to expose the starch and iodine into dark blue. Your physician will degree the amount of sweat through a clean out paper to the dark blue regions for one minute. These filter papers are then weighed to decide the rate of sweat production. This test will help decide severity of your hyperhidrosis and the response to the remedy.

Thermoregulatory Sweat Test. Your doctor may do the thermoregulatory sweat test to diagnose your hyperhidrosis. During this take a look at, your pores and pores and skin might be blanketed with a moisture-touchy powder. In the area in which there's immoderate sweating, the powder will turn from yellow-orange to darkish crimson.

In a warm temperature surroundings, someone with hyperhidrosis will tend to sweat even greater. But for the ones non-hyperhidrosis patients, they will now not sweat in the fingers. With this, your clinical physician can by means of some way effectively diagnose and description the hyperhidrosis. Your doctor may even eventually pick out the quality remedy approach perfect for you.

These quantitative diagnostic exams can substantially help in diagnosing a hyperhidrosis circumstance. It is likewise essential to apply diagnostic device to evaluate how the scenario impacts a affected man or woman's first rate of existence and the manner it distorts his or her every day sports. This can in big element effect the confirmation of the diagnosis. With this, your clinical physician can use HDSS and or distinct questionnaires.

Hyperhidrosis Disease Severity Scale (HDSS). Along with a smooth signs and signs and symptoms and signs and symptoms and signs and signs and symptoms checklist of hyperhidrosis that clinicians use, they'll moreover use a easy scale to determine the severity of your hyperhidrosis. This is known as the Hyperhidrosis Disease Severity Scale (HDSS).

The Hyperhidrosis Disease Severity Scale (HDSS) is a disease-precise, rapid, and effects-comprehended diagnostic device that gives qualitative gauge of a affected character's hyperhidrosis scenario relying on the manner it influences sports of each day dwelling (ADL). The questions within the scale may be given to the patient every thru an interview or a questionnaire.

Here is the Hyperhidrosis Disease Severity Scale (HDSS).

Your health practitioner or clinician will ask you to pick out a declaration that allows you to describe your contemporary hyperhidrosis condition. The declaration which you should select need to be the one that reflects your enjoy with sweating of the desired body aspect or region. If you could placed above, there are numbers next to the statements. These numbers will suggest how your responses can be scored.

A score of 3 or four will endorse that you have excessive hyperhidrosis. While a score of or 1 will specify moderate or moderate hyperhidrosis.

The HDSS moreover can be used yet again in placed up-treatment. It may be a manual to diploma the efficacy of the remedy that grow to be achieved and the satisfaction of the affected character. A 1 point development inside the HDSS rating will imply that there may be 50% good buy of sweat manufacturing. On the alternative hand, a 2 component reduction in the HDSS score will mean that there may be eighty% decrease within the sweat manufacturing.

Others. Your physician also can ask you severa questions like:

COMPLICATIONS

Hyperhidrosis complications are rarely medically excessive or immoderate. However, a large range of hyperhidrosis patients do enjoy a few or a mixture of those complications. Although speakme approximately the extent of annoyance or pain, immoderate perspiration or sweating may be notably off the charts. Complications of hyperhidrosis will now not high-quality consist of physiological issues, however moreover intellectual distress. While the ones complications are minor, they'll be although very important to be mentioned and given right attention and treatment.

Physiological Complications

Fungal Nail Infections. People, who generally sweat profusely like people with hyperhidrosis, are at risk or at risk of specific types of fungal infections. This is due to the truth fungi thrive in warfare and wet environments just like the inner of your sweaty footwear. That is why, it's miles very commonplace for people to have fungi infections within the toenails than in the fingernails. A fungal nail infection will generally start as a white or yellow spot under the top of your nail. As it spreads and deepens, your nail will revel in discoloration, thickening, and development of crumbling edges. Occasionally, your nail will become independent from the nail bed. The pores and skin round it will become pink and swell. Sometimes, it's far observed with the aid of moderate horrific odor.

Athlete's Foot. Athlete's foot (or medically termed as tinea pedis) is the fungal contamination of the toes. Because human beings with hyperhidrosis sweat lots, their pores and skin can be wet maximum of the time, mainly the foot. Fungus will thrive thoroughly in these moist regions. For athlete's foot, it regularly starts offevolved in some of the ft, in which profuse sweating may be extreme.

Jock Itch. Jock itch or tinea cruris is a fungal infection that takes area within the folds of the groin. The heavy or immoderate sweating inside the groin vicinity could make the area moist which can be very conducive for fungal boom.

Maceration. When your skin receives continuously wet sooner or later of heavy perspiration, the pores and skin will start to breakdown and bring about a gentle, peeling appearance.

Warts and Bacterial Infection. Due to the pores and pores and pores and skin breakdown or pores and skin maceration, it can without problems provide an get admission to for bacteria and virus to reason infections and warts.

Heat Rash. Heat rash or prickly heat takes location at the same time as the pores of the pores and skin near your sweat glands become clogged-up. It will end result to your sweat to be trapped growing purple spots or bumps on your higher returned, chest, or arms.

Body Odor. This is also called bromhidrosis. If the perfume does now not come from the sweat itself, it comes from the substances that bacteria launch while they arrive in touch with sweat. The sweat inside the underarms and the groin areas are the most probably to provide smell. Sweaty feet come 2d in phrases of fragrance produced.

There are techniques to be able to save you the ones physiological complications of hyperhidrosis. It may be mentioned inside the subsequent segment.

Psychological & Non-Physiological Complications

Social and Emotional Consequences. While for some human beings sweating isn't a trouble, human beings with hyperhidrosis deal with their excessive sweating catch 22 state of affairs very intense and incapacitating. There are many hyperhidrosis sufferers who whinge that their signs and signs and signs and signs and physiological headaches are insupportable or slightly tolerable. They avoid social contact because of the reality they may be embarrassed of the circumstance and don't need other people to comprehend the scientific trouble they're experiencing.

Educational and Occupational Consequences. Hyperhidrosis patients will in a few manner meet problems of their schooling or expert careers. For college age children and young adults, it's miles very tough for them to take part in university sports activities and to mingle with their classmates/schoolmates while they will be experiencing the signs and symptoms and symptoms of hyperhidrosis. It may be so embarrassing for them to have their buddies see them sweating excessively. On the opposite hand, adults may also revel in a few outcomes of their artwork region because of the hyperhidrosis conditions. Their paintings ethics and professionalism may be hampered and notably affected.

Chapter 4: Treatment

Hyperhidrosis can often be correctly controlled. This is so long as you'll cooperate along with your healthcare enterprise and offer him or her all of the pertinent facts about your immoderate sweating circumstance. There are a large choice of remedy techniques that your doctor will advocate or prescribe for you which of them ones is based totally completely on the severity of your hyperhidrosis.

Pharmacologic Interventions

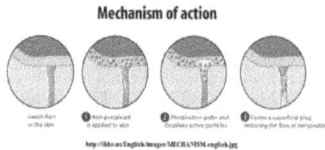

Mechanism of action

http://bbo.us/English/images/MECHANISM-english.jpg

Therapy for hyperhidrosis, particularly for its medicines, may be very hard to the affected individual and the clinical doctor as well. Topical and systemic drug remedies can be every used inside the treatment of sufferers with hyperhidrosis.

Topical Agents. If you have were given were given been identified with light to moderate hyperhidrosis, you scientific health practitioner can probably endorse so you can use or comply with non-prescription, over the counter

clinical energy antiperspirants. An antiperspirant can be implemented at the hassle areas as an initial treatment.

Most antiperspirants use aluminium slat answers. When you observe the antiperspirant, the aluminium ions are interested in the cells and water passes in with them. This will motive the cells to swell, consequently squeezing the sweat ducts close to so sweat can't get out. There are instances even as antiperspirant can even embody aluminium chloride hexahydrate. This is lots effective than aluminium, thereby very effective. Other steel salts that might paintings nicely in antiperspirants are: zirconium, indium, and vanadium.

Typically, one of the prescription antiperspirant that is cautioned as a way to use is Drysol. Drysol (20% aluminium chloride hexahydrate in absolute anhydrous ethyl alcohol) is carried out nightly on dry pores and pores and skin with or without occlusion till amazing effects are executed. Then the software program software intervals are lengthened. In order to lessen irritation, you ought to wash off the final medicinal drug from the pores and skin even as you awaken in the morning. Baking soda may be completed within the difficult region to neutralize it.

For axillary hyperhidrosis, aluminium gel can be the fine remedy. However, aluminium gel can cause mild cutaneous contamination.

Other topical entrepreneurs which have been used as remedy for hyperhidrosis consist of: topical anticholinergics, boric acid, 2%-five% tannic acid solutions, resorcinol, potassium permanganate, formaldehyde, glutaraldehyde, and methenamine. These sellers are constrained due to staining, inflammation, touch sensitization, or inadequate effectiveness. Their obstacles generally tend to make Drysol one of the first-line topical marketers for hyperhidrosis.

Agents for tanning which has astringent houses have been used for the treatment of hyperhidrosis. These sellers will denature the keratin proteins in the stratum corneum layer lining the sweat pore that consequences inside the superficial closure of the pore lasting for several days. Formaldehyde, glutaraldehyde, tannic acid, and trichloroacetic acid have also been utilized in hyperhidrosis remedy. Even despite the reality that the ones acids and aldehydes are taken into consideration out of date, there are although low concentrations of them in some commercial products.

Systemic Medications. Systemic drug treatments can be used inside the remedy of focal or generalized hyperhidrosis. Many of the drugs which might be documented to have effective or useful consequences for hyperhidrosis sufferers have now not been tested or studied in controlled trials. They are actually identified beneficial primarily based on anecdotal evidences. Moreover, side results can be restricting at high-quality doses of these systemic medicinal tablets to inhibit hyperhidrosis.

Medications for the remedy of hyperhidrosis will encompass anticholinergics. These styles of pills are first-rate as they'll inhibit the sympathetic stimulation of the eccrine glands by using the usage of using deterring the function of acetylcholine, for this reason halting sweat secretion. Antocholinergic for hyperhidrosis remedy are Propantheline bromide, Glycopyrrolate, Oxybutinin, Glycopyrronium bromide, and Benztropine.

However, the use of the ones tablets is constrained by means of the standard anticholinergic factor outcomes which includes:

•Urinary retention

•Dry mouth

•Constipation

•Visual disturbances like mydriasis, cyclopegia

If traumatic situations are the motive of the onset of hyperhidrosis, the use of an anitcholinergic agent is useful. Benzodiazipine use previous to an occasion on the manner to in all likelihood purpose anxiety or anxiety is likewise very beneficial. The long term use of benzodiazepine (which includes Diazepan) is also restricting as it can bring about the improvement of dependency or dependancy. Many patients can't moreover tolerate the overall performance of this drug as a sedative. A Diazepam dose of 5mg at bedtime for numerous weeks can be taken via some patients in reality to get use of this drug's sedating effect after which use it as vital for anxiety-frightening conditions.

On the other hand, there are uncommon instances or small range of sufferers which have recommended they've got clearly spoke back to the outcomes of numerous systemic medicines. These sufferers have unique and tremendous types of hyperhidrosis. Here are a number of the ones systemic drug remedies:

1.   Diltiazem. The use of calcium channel blocker, Diltiazem, have been mentioned to patently lessen the amount of sweating in a few sufferers with obvious autosomal dominant shape of primary focal hyperhidrosis. There are research that proposed that sweat manufacturing is in detail inspired by the use of an influx of calcium from the extracellular location of into the secretory cells of the eccrine glands. Diltiazem and specific calcium channel blocker will save you the inflow of calcium in the course of the cell membrance, thereby very beneficial in hyperhidrosis. However, there aren't any further posted reviews as to

42

hyperhidrosis remedy with calsium channel blockers.

2. Clonidine. This drug has been advised to have decreased sweating in ladies who had paroxysmal localized hyperhidrosis (that may be a uncommon scenario that may be idiopathic or because of involved device ailment, or incidence of a gustatory manifestation of sweating). With Clonidine, a affected man or woman with profuse sweating due to tricyclic antidepressant use has enjoy marked reduction in sweat manufacturing. Another report is that a person had comfort from his tension-delivered on facial and scalp hyperhidrosis after use of Clonidine and topical aluminium chloride.

3. Indomethacin. Coincidental treatment of a affected person's arthritis with Indomethacin 25 mg 3 instances a day has reduced heavy sweating. The affected man or woman had lifelong generalized hyperhidrosis that is worsening of 4-6 months and excessive night

time time sweats, however with none underlying sickness or scientific circumstance. When Indomethacin became discontinued, the affected individual's excessive sweating yet again.

4. Benztropine. A affected person with generalized hyperhidrosis (that's socially disabling) on venlafaxine spoke back to the use of anticholinergic Benztropine zero.5mg 2 instances an afternoon.

five. Oxybutynin. A affected man or woman with the uncommon syndrome of episodic hyperhidrosis with hypothermia determined comfort from his heavy sweating after being prescribed with Oxybutynin for unrelated urinary urgency. This unusual circumstance is located to be due to an abnormality of the hyporthalamus.

6. Propantheline. Often after years of spinal wire damage, patients will experience autonomic dysreflexia if you need to typically result in hyperhidrosis. There are quadriplegic sufferers had exceptional manage in their

heavy sweating with using Propantheline (an anticholinergic). They were prescribed with this drug to address neurogenic bladder (ordinary in spinal wire damage). Propantheline was anticipated to dam the cholinergic receptors that are worried in sweat production.

7. Fludrocortisone. There were patients that had cervical backbone damage and orthostatic hypotension that turn out to be belief to provoke the onset or worsen autonomic dysreflexia and hyperhidorsis. Their profuse sweating replied thoroughly once they had been treated with Fludrocortisone for their orthostatic blood stress drop.

Iontophoresis. This is the machine of passing ionized substance through intact pores and skin with the aid of the software program of a direct electric cutting-edge. Many dermatologists find out tap water iontophoresis to be the right first line of remedy for hyperhidrosis of the hands and soles. Although more awkward, iontophoresis is likewise applied in axillary hyperhidrosis. Simple tap water iontophoresis additionally can be employed to supply anticholinergics and other drug treatments to the areas which can be affected with hyperhidrosis.

The precept in the again of this treatment approach is based totally totally completely at the principle in power wherein molecules of the same price will repel, on the same time as the ones that are in some other way charged will entice. In iontophosresis, charged molecules are introduced thru the pores and skin with the useful resource of placing it close to the electrode of the identical fee, on the equal time due to the fact the electrode of the specific price is located elsewhere. However, this clarification of the manner capsules are transported through the pores and pores and skin does no longer offer an cause of the way with the resource of which tap water iontophoresis reduce sweat output. Although the mechanism of movement of tap water iontophoresis isn't always understood currently, there were numerous theories to provide an reason of the way.

The recommended recurring for iontophoresis is based upon at the device used, regions that want treatment, and whether or now not the remedy may be completed within the domestic or hospital. Here are some of the overall advices for the remedy:

•If the pores and pores and skin to be handled has scraps, cuts, or wounds, you have to cowl those with a skinny layer of petrolatum. The pores and pores and skin across the axilla place must be covered with a layer of petrolatum if treating that area.

•You should use nondeionized tap water (water from the tap).

•Only fill the trays with just enough water to cowl the fingers or ft at the same time as treating.

•After you place the region to be handled at the tray or after making use of the device or moist pads to an electrode to the axilla, you may now activate the device. You want to gradually increase the amperage till you sense a tingling sensation that isn't always uncomfortable inside the affected region or to a most of 20 mA.

•Treatment need to be for 20 mins every 2 to 3 days or for 10 mins for three to 5 instances in keeping with week. When you are midway of the 20-minute session, you need to contrary the modern-day go with the go together with the drift to exchange anode net web page on line to the opposite issue or to hold one aspect in anodal pan each consultation until euhidrosis is acquired and transfer aspects.

•You can do the palms and ft simultaneously. Just make certain that palms and feet go into separate trays.

•The frequency of the remedy will variety, however 1 to a few instances week is essential. If the mineral content fabric fabric of the tap water used is low, inadequate drift can seem. Yet, you could counteract this with the aid of manner of along with a teaspoon of baking soda to every tray.

•Pregnant ladies, humans with pacemakers, or sufferers with arrhythmias need to not be dealt with with iontophoresis. Children may be treated with iontophoresis. However, there are the ones kids that might't tolerate the equal electric powered contemporary-day utilized by adults.

•If there can be rirritation so that it will broaden alongside the water line, it may be treated with 1% hydrocortisone cream.

There are numerous side consequences which have been determined with this treatment. However, those aspect consequences are not that immoderate or extreme to prevent the remedy. Some of these outcomes may be thwarted with the resource of way of proper or appropriate education in advance than the treatment approach. To keep away from or restriction pain during the gadget, open wounds, cuts, or scraps on the pores and skin want to be protected with petrolatum. Education and right know-how of the machine and tool will save you mid shocks.

There are some of patients handled with iontophoresis exhibited sure facet outcomes. Although typically temporary, vesiculation has been determined inside the affected regions. Redness of the pores and skin along the water line is likewise a common endorsed factor effect. Aside from erythema, pain (burning sensation or 'pins and needles') is also a commonplace criticism.

Erythema and vesiculation can be treated with 1% hydrocortisone cream if these signs and symptoms insist. The use of moisturizers or the lower of the frequency of the remedy is the treatment for dry, cracked, or fissured pores and pores and skin.

Botulinum Toxin Injections (Botox). Botulinum Injection A has been located to be very a success in in decresing the heaving perspiration in the frame areas laid low with number one hyperhidrosis much like the palmoplantar, axlllary, and facial/gustatory regions. This minimally invasive remedy is essentially recommended for hyperhidrosis sufferers who have now not surely replied to the conservative healing techniques. Botulinum toxin A has been approved to be used as a hyperhidrosis treatment in many nations on the facet of Canada, the United Kingdom, and distinctive worldwide locations in Europe and South America (extra than 23 international locations in universal). The US Food and Drug Administration has given acclaim for Botulinum Toxin A to be used for sufferers with number one hyperhidrosis that has not replied when they used antiperspirants.

Generally, Botox injections are not appropriate for men and women who're allergic to it. For the ones sufferers with neuromuscular illness, contamination on the injection internet internet web page, and people who're taking antibiotics and any other medicinal tablets that may disrupt with

51

the neuromuscular transmission, Botox injections need to no longer receive.

Before the Botox may be injected, a topical anesthetic can be given to the region to be treated. This will prevent the pain from the multiple injections wished at some level within the treatment. When the region is dry, Botox is injected proper now on your sweat glands in the treatment region. Usually, it takes 15 to 20 injections using a totally fin needle each treatment consultation. The Botox is injected below the pores and pores and skin. It will take 15 minutes for every consultation. There is mild ache inside the remedy region at some stage within the injections.

After the remedy, there are a few people who will revel in a few pain and bleeding in the remedy region. Side outcomes will embody heavy sweating outside the treatment area, headache, fever, sore throat, itching, neck and returned pain, and tension. Once the Botox will take impact, you need now not use underarm dress or blouse guard. You can also switch from prescription antiperspirant to non-prescription antiperspirant.

The sweat discount in Botox Injections isn't always eternal. The remedy will usually want to copy for six to 8 months sincerely so that you can preserve its results. You can be aware the full-size discount in your immoderate perspiration interior 4 weeks of your remedy. If you don not have any marked splendid outcomes, you should need to the touch your healthcare agency and ask for a look at-up consultation.

Surgical Interventions

When all distinct treatment techniques were tried and adjusted for fine occasions however didn't pretty offer the incredible results, surgical treatments for hyperhidrosis need to be quality taken into consideration via way of your healthcare company. There are one-of-a-type forms of surgical remedy that can be decided on through way of your health practitioner to find consolation out of your profuse perspiration catch 22 situation. These encompass the neighborhood surgical removal of the sweat glands, Endosopic Thoracic Sympathectomy (ETS), and Endosopic Lumbar Sympathectomy (ELS).

Local Surgical Techniques. This is known as as close by due to the reality the manner is completed on the location or factor of sweating. The neighborhood strategies of sweat gland suction and excision, retrodermal curettage, and axillary liposuction may be finished with a purpose to cope with immoderate underarm perspiration. During the excision, the sweat glands can be eliminated or reduce out. The retrodermal curettage implies that the sweat glands are scraped out. Axillary liposuction eliminates 30% of the sweat glands, as a result main to the proportionate bargain of sweat manufacturing. These are what dermatologists frequently propose as network surgical techniques as effects are promising.

Endosopic Thoracic Sympathectomy (ETS). This manner has been hooked up to have reduced the excessive amount of perspiration a number of the bulk of sufferers with hyperhidrosis. However, there are a few clinical medical docs who're having 2d mind of recommending this approach to their hyperhidrosis sufferers. Yet, the excessive pleasure fees of sufferers who've long past via this manner has established that it's far very powerful and stable.

This way is aimed in the direction of interrupting the transmission of nerve signs and symptoms from the spinal wire to the sweat glands. When this is interrupted, the sympathetic fearful gadget will now not have the capability of "turning on" the sweat glands of your frame. The thoracic or chest medical doctor will reduce, burn, or clamp the thoracic ganglion at the primary sympathetic chain that runs alongside the spinal cord. Once the sympathetic chain is disrupted, the heavy or profuse sweating is long past. The results are pretty proper now.

ETS is commonly taken into consideration to be a stable and effective system. Many patients are satisfied with the effects of the surgical remedy. Reports have demonstrated that satisfaction fees pass over eighty% and plenty better in pediatric sufferers. This approach will provide treatment 85% to ninety 5% of sufferers with palmar hyperhidrosis. This also may be beneficial in axillary hyperhidrosis. Although this will moreover be for people who enjoy facial blushing and facial sweating, there are quite a few times that have been a failure. Some of these patients will experience undesirable factor results. But, it has no longer been established in controlled trials but.

After the surgery, maximum human beings can get higher at home after spending some hours enhancing from the anesthesia in the sanatorium. Under maximum situations, entire recuperation might be carried out after some days.

Compensatory sweating is the primary side impact after present system ETS. It is the heavy sweating on the chest, all over again, stomach, legs, face, and buttocks. This can be a very extreme difficulty effect because the sweating may be in addition or more immoderate than the unique sweating seize 22 situation of the affected individual. Other element results embody hemothorax (blood in the thoracic hollow area, within the again of the lungs) and recurrence of signs.

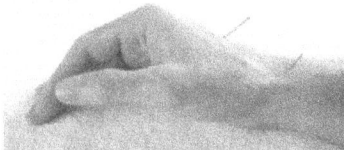

http://www.prevent-sweating.com/graphics/acupuncture.gif

Knowing the side effects, you need to undergo in mind them earlier than you choose ETS. You and your health practitioner need to have exhausted all the possible remedies (non-surgical) in advance than touchdown on the selection for surgical operation. Make positive that you have explored the to be had remedy like prescription-electricity antiperspirants, systemic drug treatments, botox injections, iontophoresis, and the mixture of numerous those treatments.

Lumbar Sympathectomy. This is a exceedingly new surgical operation for humans who have now not discovered comfort after ETS for their plantar hyperhidrosis. In this procedure, the sympathetic chain at the lumbar region is clipped or divided that allows you to allay immoderate and profuse foot sweating. Ninety percentage is mentioned to be the achievement charge. Patients are given this feature after they (affected person and medical doctor) have exhausted all conservative treatment strategies.

If you're approximately to keep in thoughts the surgical interventions, you need to invite your physician to offer you with the complete facts about the approach. If possible, ask your scientific medical doctor to tell you what he goes to do. Knowing the risks and aspect consequences also will let you're making a valid choice in case you need to push thru with any of the techniques referred to.

Other Treatment Methods

You may additionally moreover have heard of various hyperhidrosis sufferers who are present process numerous opportunity treatment strategies to alleviate their extreme sweating disaster. There are natural substances which may be said to help in hyperhidrosis. These are sage tea or sage capsules, chamomile, valerian root, St. John's Wort, and tea tree oil. Other techniques which is probably suggested to offer capability remedy for hyperhidrosis are acupuncture, biofeedback, hypnosis, and relation techniques. Today, these kinds of opportunity treatment interventions have little studies to once more up their effectiveness, but this doesn't make their functionality to deal with plenty much less massive and beneficial.

Herbal Substances. There are positive herbal plant life or materials that may be used for the remedy of hyperhidrosis. However, in advance than you take any of those herbal preparations, you ought to speak to your doctor regarding possible side effects, appropriate dosage, and capacity drug interplay. Just keep in mind to constantly exercising caution because of the fact you don't want your immoderate and spontaneous sweating to get worse.

1. Sage. Also known as Salvia officinalis, Sage is a member of the mint own family, it really is a perennial evergreen shrub that grows within the Mediterranean. Today, it furthermore grows in North America. It has a aromatic odor and a smelly flavor this is said to have drying and warming dispositions. Aside from medicinal capabilities, it's also employed for culinary use. The aerial herb at its budding diploma is used to make the pharmaceutical guidance. Sage is an effective natural treatment for spontaneous sweating, in particular for night time time sweats. This

natural remedy has astringent and carminative homes that help to test heavy perspiration, heat flashes, night time time sweats, and mucuous membrane inflammation. Pregnant girls are not endorsed to take sage as this could stimulate menstruation.

Chapter 5: Lifestyle Changes & Home Remedies

When you be bothered with the resource of hyperhidrosis, you may locate that there may be some factor out of your life-style that must be blamed. Making some few changes will no longer remedy your hyperhidrosis, but it'll come what may additionally additionally improve your flailing self warranty and vanity. Some manner of lifestyles modifications can provide ease of signs and signs and symptoms and (in a few instances) will provide you with a marked improvement on your today's fitness.

Remember, a number of the ones changes had been said within the PREVENTION segment of this eBook. In addition, these hints are not treatment in your excessive sweating lure 22 state of affairs.

Nutrition

There are foods and drinks which you want to keep away from in order no longer to result in excessive perspiration or sweating. On the opportunity hand, there are folks that permit you to along side your heavy sweating disaster.

Let us start with those which you need to keep away from.

AVOID...

Garlic. The garlic's robust sulfur compounds are metabolized which incorporates allyl methyl sulfide. Allyl Methyl Sulfide (AMS) can't be digested, but is handed into the blood pass. It is then carried to the lungs and excreted through the pores and pores and skin. Thus, it'll hasten the production of sweat.

Onions. The pungency of onions has a heating impact that may increase the blood circulate. This will increase the body temperature, thereby reason the sweating. This form of effect will decrease down fevers and sweat out flu and colds. However, for hyperhidrosis sufferers, this impact will certainly get worse the state of affairs.

Caffeine. Caffeine is decided in numerous generally consumed gadgets like colas, electricity drinks, espresso, tea, cocoa, chocolate, weight reduction aids, prescription and non-prescription medicinal drugs. The link amongst sweating and caffeine is in fact apparent. Caffeine is a sturdy stimulant which can improve your body middle temperature, enhance blood pressure, increase waft and heartbeat.

Spicy Food. Peppers and tremendous highly spiced dishes can accelerate your metabolism, consequently increasing the sweat manufacturing. Its impact is much like that of caffeine.

Alcohol. Initially, alcohol can dehydrate your frame. When you drink, you can possibly visit the relaxation room too frequently. However, that is though the first degree. In some time, your center frame temperature will improve that may motive the acceleration of fluids to be flushed from your frame through your pores and pores and skin pores.

CONSUME...

Water. Some hyperhidrosis patients assume that the greater they drink water, the extra they may sweat. Actually, ingesting cool or cold water can decrease your frame temperature. When your inner frame temperature is beneath manipulate, your sweating can be saved at bay.

Sage Tea. As you've got were given observe inside the previous phase, sage is includes astringent houses. Sage tea is diagnosed as a natural antiperspirant that prevents sweating inner out. It is a systemic approach in controlling your hyperhidrosis circumstance.

Fruits. Aside from exceedingly very wholesome, culmination may be a super assist inside the control of the heavy perspiration. Mostly, fruits comprise 80% water that could truly make a contribution to the cooling impact that your body desires.

Olive Oil. Apart from being a wholesome fats that decreases ldl ldl cholesterol and reduces blood pressure, olive oil can be an remarkable replacement to wonderful forms of oil in your food. The strength to digest olive oil is an entire lot a lot less, thus reducing the need for the frame to exert and burn up power.

Whole Grains. The actual thriller of entire grains is they contain masses of B vitamins. These nutrients can allow your frame to characteristic effectively, requiring much less try and power. With less attempt and electricity, there also can be plenty much less warmth this is produced inner your frame- for that reason an entire lot lots much less sweating for you.

CLOTHING

"What to position on?" – that is really one of the equal vintage each day dilemma of hyperhidrosis patients. You may additionally moreover have professional (along facet numerous hyperhidrosis patients) having to stare for a couple of minutes at your closet each morning to discover the great and "maximum stable" garb to vicinity on that might be appropriate for the climate and the possibility of an onset of heavy sweating happens. Choosing the proper apparel to position on is a key factor in the way of life of hyperhidrosis patients.

The first to deal with is the undergarments. There are pretty some options of undergarments for each males and females who're stricken by hyperhidrosis. Find undergarments that might supply a superb safety. If you do, you could truely placed on a greater diversity of colours and cloth.

Hyperhidrosis patients ought to keep in mind some big factors in terms of apparel. Dark colored shirts and blouses are the least to show sweat marks. Knitted fabric and "sweater" fabric in any material content material material can soak up sweat, because of this a great deal much less sweat marks. Jackets, blazers, and cardigans can cowl-up sweat, but (lamentably) can exacerbate your state of affairs as it could motive you to overheat and sweat extra. Clothing with patterns are super at protecting or concealing sweat.

If you are uncertain whether or not or no longer a effective material of a garb you are attempting to shop for at a department maintain, you could do a water bottle take a look at. In the fine room, you can placed some drops of water on the garment and notice what takes region. There are garments wherein they soak up right now the water, others don't. There are also some cloth in which water will simply roll off.

Personal Hygiene

Because you comprehend you'll sweat nearly all day and in all likelihood produce body scent, ordinary bathing for two to three instances an afternoon can be beneficial. This isn't only to take away frame scent, but additionally to dispose of bacteria. You can use a cleaning soap this is advocated for your clinical condition. Although this may now not actually do away with your hyperhidrosis, going for walks toward proper and regular non-public hygiene will can help you growth your shallowness and self assurance. Aside from that, you may additionally control your frame temperature thru showering or taking a shower.

After bathing, dry thoroughly all of the regions of your body, in particular those areas affected most of your hyperhidrosis situation. Dry your armpits and feet very well. You must change your shoes alternately to permit them to dry. Never wear the same socks the following day. Wear socks which is probably crafted from natural fabric.

Chapter 6: Sweating Basics

What is Sweat?

Sweating (or "perspiration") is the release of a salty liquid from the body's sweat glands. Once the sweat is at the pores and pores and skin floor, evaporation of the sweat makes the skin cooler and allows the body maintain its temperature. Thus, sweat affords a very critical mechanism to protect frame from overheating.

Interestingly, mammals are the best animal organization able to sweating, and there are specific mechanisms used by non-mammals, in addition to mammals to hold themselves cooler (e.G. Puppies pant to hold themselves cool, and hippos immerse themselves in water).

Coming once more to humans (the enterprise I suspect you're most interested by): Sweat comes out through sweat glands dispensed throughout our frame. A general human frame has about to 4 million sweat glands.

Two Types of Sweat Glands

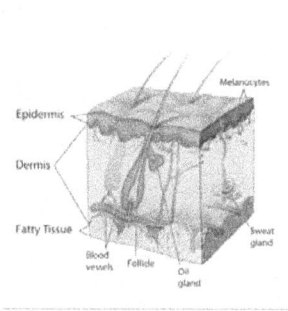

There are 2 kinds of sweat glands:

Most of those glands are what are called "eccrine" sweat glands and are observed in huge numbers, often at the arms, the soles, the forehead and cheeks, and inside the armpits. These glands secrete an odorless, clear fluid that facilitates the body to control its temperature through the usage of selling heat loss thru evaporation. In well-known, the shape of sweat worried in excessive sweating situations (hyperhidrosis) is eccrine sweat.

The unique sort of sweat gland is referred to as an "apocrine" gland. Apocrine glands are found in the armpits and genital place. They produce a thick fluid. When this fluid comes in contact with micro organism at the pores and skin's floor, it produces a feature robust "frame odor".

How We Sweat?

Sweating is managed through manner of the autonomic nervous gadget, the a part of the involved system that isn't always underneath your manage. This ensures that the body is capable of maintaining its temperature with none energetic attempt from the individual. Because sweating is the frame's natural manner of regulating temperature, human beings sweat more whilst it's heat outdoor. In addition to cooling off goals, human beings moreover sweat extra after they exercise, or in response to situations that cause them to fearful, angry, embarrassed, or afraid. These nerves respond to pretty some stimuli collectively with:

Heat: When thoughts signs and symptoms that the frame may be liable to overheating, sweat glands come into movement to carry the temperature down

Anxiety associated emotions (e.G. Frightened, irritated, afraid and plenty of others.): When faced with a demanding situation, our adrenal gland release hormones which includes adrenaline. This hormone triggers sweat glands as it is also the hormone that prepares frame for any forthcoming war of terms (e.G. Attacked through an animal): the schooling consist of making frame cool for the approaching war of words.

hormones (e.G. At some stage in menopause)

Physical pastime or exercise: When the frame is workout, it releases a number of warm temperature. This triggers the body's reaction to launch sweat to carry the temperature down yet again.

When the sweat gland is stimulated, the cells secrete a fluid this is largely water and it has immoderate concentrations of sodium and chloride and a low interest of potassium. This fluid comes from the areas a number of the cells, which in flip receives the fluid from the blood vessels near the skin. While the fluid is passing via the ducts, relying upon the sweat volumes, this form of seem:

Low sweat manufacturing (e.G. Cool temperature): The fluid travels slowly, consequently cells within the duct have sufficient time to reabsorb maximum of the sodium and chlorine from the fluid. Thus, by the time sweat oozes at the pores and pores and pores and skin, there isn't always as masses sodium and chloride, and there's greater potassium.

High sweat manufacturing (e.G. Exercise) - The fluid travels rapid, and the cells within the duct do no longer have enough time to reabsorb all of sodium and chloride from the primary secretion. So, some of sweat makes it to the ground of the pores and skin and the sodium and chloride focus are better.

Sweat is produced in apocrine sweat glands in the equal way. However, the sweat from apocrine glands additionally incorporates proteins and fatty acids, which make it thicker and supply it a milkier or yellowish coloration (the purpose why underarm stains in clothing appear yellowish). Sweat itself has no heady scent, but on the equal time as bacteria at the pores and skin and hair metabolize the proteins and fatty acids, they produce an unsightly scent. This is why deodorants and anti-perspirants are finished to the underarms in desire to the entire body.

Chapter 7: Excessive Sweating

I am frightened due to the fact I am sweating, not sweating due to the truth I am worried!

Introduction to Hyperhidrosis

As mentioned in final financial disaster, sweating is an important mechanism to adjust body temperature. However, for a few human beings, this mechanism is overactive – i.E. The character sweats a first-rate deal greater than it's miles vital to regulate the temperature and on occasion even with none of the equal vintage triggers (heat, anxiety, anxiety and so forth.).

Hyperhidrosis is a noticeably common state of affairs, specifically given the shortage of facts approximately this sickness. An expected 3% of population (i.E. About 7.Five million humans in US, greater than one hundred and 80 million people global) suffers with a few shape of hyperhidrosis. That manner that during case you're a mean Facebook patron with approximately 350 friends, opportunities are that approximately 10 of these Facebook pals have a few form of hyperhidrosis! And you concept you have been by myself?

Measuring Hyperhidrosis

There are numerous techniques which may be used to degree the severity of hyperhidrosis. Gravimetry and evaporimetry are carried out in scientific research to degree the amount of the sweat. However, such tests aren't realistic in non-studies setting, and rather self-evaluation questionnaires are used that degree the impact of hyperhidrosis on affected person's splendid of life to determine the severity of hyperhidrosis.

Hyperhidrosis Impact Questionnaire (HHIQ) is a questionnaire in particular designed to diploma the severity of Hyperhidrosis.. HHIQ has questions for baseline evaluation, in addition to questions for study-up remedy. However, that is complicated and is commonly utilized in research settings simplest.

A sensible degree for measuring hyperhidrosis severity this is often used is the Hyperhidrosis Disease Severity Scale (HDSS). HDSS gives a qualitative measure of the severity of the affected person's situation based totally on the way it influences every day sports activities. This is a deceptively clean questionnaire wherein the sufferers pick out the announcement that awesome displays their enjoy with sweating within the positive place. Each alternative has a score among 1 to 4. A score of three or 4 indicates intense hyperhidrosis, at the same time as a score of one or 2 suggests moderate or slight primary hyperhidrosis.

HDSS allows doctors to choose out the impact of hyperhidrosis on affected person's each day sports activities activities. HDSS has been verified to have very sturdy correlations to extra complex methods of measuring the severity of hyperhidrosis, and is as a result a legitimate degree. A 1-issue improvement in HDSS score is related to a 50% discount in sweat production, at the same time as a 2-point development with an 80% cut charge

To get your Hyperhidrosis Disease Severity Scale (HDSS), solution the following query

"How could you rate the severity of your hyperhidrosis?"

1.My sweating is in no way amazing and in no way interferes with my each day sports

2.My sweating is tolerable however every so often interferes with my each day sports activities activities

three.My sweating is slightly tolerable and frequently interferes with my every day sports

4.My sweating is insupportable and constantly interferes with my each day sports activities

Your score is the variety related to the chosen preference. For example, if you made a decision on the choice "My sweating is tolerable but every so often interferes with

my every day sports", your HDSS rating is —
i.E. Moderate hyperhidrosis.

As regular with a check finished in 2004, the
split of Hyperhidrosis patients thru the usage

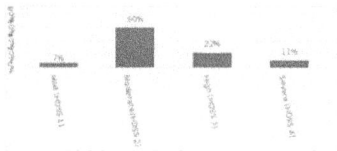

of their HDSS rating is as follows.

Thus, multiple 0.33 of hyperhidrosis patients
have immoderate to intense hyperhidrosis.
Taking the example above, which means that
about 3 of your Facebook friends have
hyperhidrosis this is severe sufficient to
intrude with their every day lives. You already
revel in better – don't you?

Types of Hyperhidrosis

Hyperhidrosis may have an effect on a
particular body factors, or the overall body.
Palms, toes, underarm, and the groin are
maximum common areas impacted with the

useful resource of Hyperhidrosis. For some motive, clinical professionals like to name them via more complex names, and it's beneficial to understand the clinical phrases of your Hyperhidrosis. Following are the essential thing forms of hyperhidrosis. Please word that the severa varieties of hyperhidrosis aren't together one-of-a-kind – human beings can (and regularly) suffer from hyperhidrosis in more than one frame factors.

General vs. Primary Focal Hyperhidrosis

General Hyperhidrosis is a condition whilst the more sweating occurs at some point of the body and isn't always limited to any unique body issue. This form of hyperhidrosis can frequently be a secondary hyperhidrosis (i.E. Caused thru an underlying scientific circumstance) – however, that isn't always continuously the case.

Primary Focal Hyperhidrosis is on the same time as a selected body element suffers from immoderate sweating, and isn't always a end cease end result of a few unique underlying situation. This is the form of hyperhidrosis we will trouble ourselves with for most detail on this e-book for the cause that General Hyperhidrosis is often handled through managing the underlying scientific condition.

Palmar Hyperhidrosis

Palmar Hyperhidrosis is the medical time period for the hyperhidrosis imp acting hands (frequently fingers). This is one of the maximum commonplace kinds of hyperhidrosis, and in all likelihood the best that impact the social existence the most. Persons having Palmar Hyperhidrosis frequently have problem in managing the crucial social interactions which encompass shaking hands or protecting hands. It may additionally moreover cause greater practical troubles like maintaining gadget or guidance wheel or a pen for that depend.

Plantar Hyperhidrosis

Palmar Hyperhidrosis is the medical term for the hyperhidrosis impacting ft (normally soles). People tormented by this sort of hyperhidrosis sweat on their ft. While this type of hyperhidrosis is tons much less tough to cover beneath shoes/socks, it's miles despite the truth that a hard state of affairs as it could make the feet slippery.

Axillary Hyperhidrosis

Axillary hyperhidrosis is the clinical time period for hyperhidrosis centered inside the underarm region. Underarm are has the best attention of sweat glands at the frame and maximum of the humans sweat closely on this place on the equal time as doing physical interest (e.G. Walking). People with Axillary Hyperhidrosis sweat from underarm areas even without any motive. People with Axillar hyperhidrosis usually show a sweat patch on their shirts/t-shirts and might become self-conscious and disturbing in social settings because of this.

Chapter 8: Hyperhidrosis

"All we understand continues to be infinitely a good deal less than all that remains unknown" - William Harvey

Here is the lowest-line, regardless of what all of us tells you: In-spite of all the clinical advances, we're yet to understand exactly why some people be troubled with the aid of immoderate sweating. However, there are some less costly theories:

Underlying Medical Condition

Secondary hyperhidrosis is attributable to an underlying clinical circumstance. This sort of hyperhidrosis is can begin at any difficulty in existence, commonly in maturity. While the whole listing of underlying reasons continues to be now not appeared, the subsequent situations had been located to be associated with hyperhidrosis:

Menopause

Pregnancy

Thyroid issues

Diabetes

Alcoholism

Infectious illnesses like tuberculosis

Parkinson's disease

Rheumatoid arthritis

Stroke

Heart failure

Cancers like leukemia and lymphoma

This form of hyperhidrosis commonly disappears after the underlying scientific condition is resolved.

Genetics

Primary or focal hyperhidrosis normally starts offevolved offevolved throughout teens or maybe in advance than, and is thought to be inherited as a dominant genetic trait. As in line with one observe[i], approximately one-0.33 of hyperhidrosis patients had a own family data of the infection. Another look at positioned the variety at almost -1/3[ii].

The method of passing on hyperhidrosis is thought to be autosomal dominant mode (a shape of genetic inheritance) – essentially which means that there's approximately 1 in 2 risk of a parent having the hyperhidrosis gene passing it to their children (if exceptional one of the discern has the affected gene).

Not definitely all and sundry who has the gene shows symptoms of Hyperhidrosis. It is notion that about 5% of the populace includes the hyperhidrosis genes, even though best 3% of them show the signs and symptoms. However, someone who apparently does not suffer from hyperhidrosis may also in truth skip alongside the scenario to their offspring. This may additionally moreover moreover provide an motive for those people having hyperhidrosis that do not appear to have any history of the state of affairs of their instant circle of relatives.

If you've got hyperhidrosis, bypass looking for your prolonged circle of relatives and check if everybody else has a similar scenario. This is less complex than stated as hyperhidrosis isn't an brazenly stated circumstance, and once in a while even the instantaneous own family members do no longer comprehend if a person has an immoderate sweat trouble.

Chapter 9: How Hyperhidrosis Impacts Life

Often trivialized (what some sweat in the long run!), Hyperhidrosis has very real and excessive effect on the nice of life. True it does now not kill you, or incapacitates - however, the circumstance can severely limit the affected person's ability to live a extremely good lifestyles – socially, psychologically and physical.

Social Impact of Hyperhidrosis

Hyperhidrosis sufferers, especially those stricken by hyperhidrosis within the body components that are not hidden in the again of clothes frequently go through embarrassing social conditions – resulting in avoidance of social interactions, low self warranty in social situations or worse low vanity.

Shaking Hands – For humans struggling with palmar hyperhidrosis, even the simple undertaking of shaking fingers with others in social or commercial agency settings is a daunting task. A clammy handshake is often appeared to be impersonal/cold or perhaps a signal of anxiety. Many hyperhidrosis sufferers are appeared to be a good deal much less confident in interview situations because of a sweaty handshake.

Holding Hands- Holding fingers is a everyday, expected conduct among couples and lets in convey the couple collectively. However, palmar hyperhidrosis patients are often very conscious of their sweaty fingers and avoid retaining their loved ones fingers. This also can have excessive impact on the exceptional of relationship.

Public appearance- Any public appearance brings in extra tension and pressure. While maximum humans can cowl their anxiety, it's written anywhere inside the face and/or underarms of patients struggling with facial or axillary hyperhidrosis. As a cease result they get even more irritating and privy to how they're being perceived ensuing in even greater sweat.

Wearing positive clothing & accessories – Hyperhidrosis sufferers have to often do not forget their condition whilst selecting apparel. Many patients keep away from sporting slight solar sunglasses as they will be inclined to get stained with underarm sweat, similarly to avoid carrying sleeveless clothing that makes the underarm sweat visible. Similarly, girls suffering with plantar hyperhidrosis might also avoid sporting open sandals.

Perception of being un-hygienic-Hyperhidrosis has no longer some factor to do with non-public hygiene. However, hyperhidrosis sufferers are frequently considered as un-hygienic by manner of different humans because of the seen sweat on the frame and the sweat trail left on chairs, glass counters and so forth.

Practical Impact of Hyperhidrosis

Apart from the impact of hyperhidrosis on the social interactions, hyperhidrosis also can constrain the affected character's potential/effectiveness at doing a little regular responsibilities

Ability to maintain device – Severe sorts of palmar hyperhidrosis can limit one's capability to preserve sure tools tightly and for this reason also can furthermore result in a ability chance for self and others. This may additionally result in an awful lot much less interest possibilities or growth capacity for hyperhidrosis sufferers in terrific activity profiles (e.G. Production)

Writing on paper – Palmar hyperhidrosis can purpose immoderate issues with writing on paper because the paper has a unethical to get wet below the hand, ensuing in a smudged writing. This is specifically actual in excessive strain examinations conditions wherein the patients sweat more than regular.

Driving – Many hyperhidrosis sufferers discover maintaining the steering wheel a frightening challenge due to excessive sweat at the fingers. This can be particularly dangerous in conditions wherein the patients' desires to stress for extended hours, or even as the the usage of is also related to strain (e.G. Truck the usage of)

Psychological Impact of Hyperhidrosis

However, the most devastating effect of immoderate sweat is mental. Hyperhidrosis can result in low self perception, frustration or worse despair.

Loss of self assurance – Patients with extreme hyperhidrosis have issues appearing the handiest of obligations, or retaining ordinary social relationships (see the above sections). This can bring about lack of self notion, particularly on the same time as different human beings of their social circles have terrible information of hyperhidrosis and as a result can't provide a supportive surroundings.

Frustration - Chronic sweating and lack of functionality to have ordinary social interactions can bring about the affected person feeling helpless and annoyed.

Depression – In excessive instances, prolonged untreated hyperhidrosis may even bring about scientific despair because the patient may not even understand that it's a clinical situation

Chapter 10: Treatments For Hyperhidrosis

A little more staying power, a hint greater try, and what regarded hopeless failure may moreover flip to first rate achievement.

Bad information first: there may be no mentioned remedy for Hyperhidrosis. That makes experience if you hold in mind that we

don't' actually apprehend what reasons it in the first region.

However, that hasn't stopped a whole enterprise of unscrupulous operators in search of to make a brief greenback driving on the tension of Hyperhidrosis sufferers. In this bankruptcy, we're capable of have a look at the severa remedies for dealing with hyperhidrosis which have been scientifically mounted to work. Note that now not all treatment alternatives are appropriate for anyone - so that you will but want to decide out what will come up with the effects you need, however I desire this could come up with with a excessive diploma panorama of the hyperhidrosis remedy alternatives that allows you to come to be aware about the fake from real.

Broadly speakme, there are four training of remedy options for Hyperhidrosis. Yes, that many! However earlier than you get too excited, recognise that not all remedies are suitable for every person and also you want to do your studies and consult an authorized professional to select which one is first rate for you.

Treatment CategoryTreatment

TraditionalAntiperspirant

Oral remedy

Specialized non invasiveIontophoresis

MiraDry

Botox

SurgeryEndoscopic thoracic sympathectomy (ETS)

Local underarm surgical procedure

AlternativeDiet Control

Herbs

Acupuncture

Hypnosis

Antiperspirants

Antiperspirants are of-course the first line of defense towards immoderate sweat. Not best they are with out troubles to be had, they are moreover rate powerful and convenient with very little thing impact. However, the notable print is that the ones might not artwork for extreme hyperhidrosis, and the effects are quick - for this reason wanting each day software.

Commonly seemed antiperspirants are resultseasily available over the counter in most pharmacies/grocery stores. High electricity antiperspirants, which have a higher interest of aluminum oxide, are also available at pharmacies. Very excessive strength antiperspirants are typically to be had handiest through a prescription, but your dermatologist can offer you with a prescription (or maybe better, a loose pattern)

How antiperspirants paintings?

The maximum vital "active" thing in all antiperspirants is aluminum primarily based totally completely. This aluminum-based compound can also consists of severa one-of-a-type styles of aluminum which includes Aluminum chlorohydrate, Aluminum chloride, Aluminum hydroxybromide, Aluminum Sesquichlorohydrateor Aluminum zicronium tricholorohydrex glycine, in addition to many others.

When an antiperspirant is executed to the pores and skin it prevents or blocks sweat from achieving the floor of the pores and skin, because of this decreasing undesired sweat. Once an antiperspirant is achieved to the pores and skin, perspiration inside the underarm grabs and dissolves the antiperspirant particles, pulling them into the pores and forming superficial plugs which may be simply beneath the floor of the pores and pores and skin. When the body senses that the sweat duct is plugged, a comments mechanism stops the go with the flow. The plugs can stay in area at least 24 hours after which can be washed away through the years.

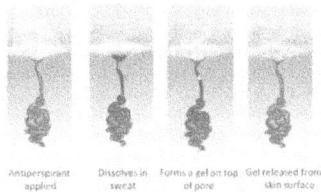

Antiperspirant applied   Dissolves in sweat   Forms a gel on top of pore   Gel released from skin surface

Regular Antiperspirants vs. High strength anti-perspirants

While you can start with the usage of a everyday antiperspirant inside the affected place, those do now not typically offer superb consolation from immoderate sweat. There are several stronger (scientific electricity) and specialised antiperspirants for hyperhidrosis that can be more effective. There are a large style of medical electricity antiperspirant brands to be had within the marketplace, every with multiple alternatives in phrases of power and shape. Many of actually high power antiperspirants for hyperhidrosis can also moreover additionally require a prescription in positive markets, on the identical time as others with a lower energy (however plenty higher than the ordinary ones) are available over the counter.

In USA, the FDA allows over the counter sale of antiperspirants containing 15%-25% aluminum (with the figure diverse based on the precise compound getting used).

One thing to study is that Antiperspirants for hyperhidrosis are normally greater powerful for the underarm region (in evaluation to palms, feet or face). This is on the complete due to the reality the pores and pores and pores and skin on fingers and toes is a high-quality deal thicker than armpits, consequently making absorption of antiperspirant trickier.

Popular over the counter antiperspirants for hyperhidrosis

In stylish, maximum over-the-counter antiperspirants include a few shape of aluminum based compound as being the principle active component (even though there are a few exceptions) – normally aluminum chloride or aluminum chlorohydrate. However, those compounds can also bring about pores and skin contamination, so wonderful compounds were gaining recognition in modern years (e.G. Aluminum zirconium tetrachlorohydrex glycine). Nevertheless, Aluminum Chloride remains the most famous compound in most OTC antiperspirants.

The following desk summarizes the most well-known antiperspirants to be had over the counter in USA. If those do now not be virtually right for you, your scientific health practitioner may moreover moreover prescribe a better strength antiperspirant as properly.

BrandFormsCompound

Certain DriRoll on, Solid, PadsAluminum chloride (15%)

OdabanSpray, LotionAluminum chloride (20%)

DrysolDab on, SolutionAluminum chloride (20%)

DriclorRoll-on, SolutionAluminum chloride (20%)

SweatBlockWipesAluminum chloride (14%)

DoveSolidAluminum zirconium Tetrachlorohydrex gly (20%)

CarpeLotionAluminum Sesquichlorohydrate (15%)

Side Effects of Antiperspirants for Hyperhidrosis

Antiperspirants are normally secure (until you have any precise response to them);. However, aluminum chloride (a common ingredient) may also additionally motive slight to mild pores and pores and skin inflammation. Some of the excessive strength antiperspirants can also make skin extraordinarily dry and itchy. The issue-outcomes, in maximum instances are quite moderate and reversible.

Oral Medication

A certified clinical professional can prescribe you a treatment plan that stops the stimulation of the sweat glands. While such drug treatments often have undesirable aspect impact, especially for long time utilization, they'll be taken into consideration underneath superb situations:

If the affected man or woman has attempted topical remedies (antiperspirants, Botox, Iontophoresis) unsuccessfully

If the hyperhidrosis affects body additives that aren't amenable to the topical remedies (e.G. Scalp, groin, genitals etc.)

If the affected individual suffers from compensatory sweating put up an ETS surgical operation

There are severa classes of medicinal drugs, relying on the ideal scenario of the affected person. Some of the vital instructions of medication used to cope with hyperhidrosis embody anxiolytics, anti-cholinergics and antimuscarinics, beta-blockers and antihypertensives.

Anxiolytics

Anxiolytic is a term carried out to all medicines that act on the thoughts, and make the affected character plenty less disturbing and traumatic. Examples of Anxiolytics include Diazepam, Alprazolam and citalopram. These pills are powerful in instances in which immoderate sweating is due to anxiety, fear or nervousness.

Beta blockers

Along with Anxiolytics, sufferers with tension may additionally discover beta-blockers beneficial for stress-brought about hyperhidrosis. Beta-blockers block adrenaline and one-of-a-kind substances that make us stressful, as a end result making us lots less probably to sweat. Unlike Anxiolytics, they act on the nerve device and no longer the mind, and are not needed to be taken often.

Antihypertensives

Antihypertensives are a class of medicine which might be used to treat high blood pressure. However it has moreover been determined effective at treating hyperhidrosis. Clonidine, a shape of Antihypertensive, reduces stimulation of the nerves which allow sweating, hence lowering the quantity of sweat.

Anti-cholinergics

Anti-chlorinergics capsules are typically prescribed for a big type of other conditions, collectively with urinary problems or an overactive bladder. Long time period use of Anti-cholinergics is not advocated for hyperhidrosis due to doubtlessly excessive aspect results. Some of the compounds beneath this elegance embody Robinul

(Glycopyrromium Bromide), Oxybutynin (Ditropan), Pro-Banthine (Propantheline Bromide)

Iontophoresis

What is Iontophoresis

Iontophoresis is a drug shipping method that makes use of a small electric powered powered charge to supply the drug through the pores and skin – almost like an injection, however without a needle. For hyperhidrosis remedy, Iontophoresis is finished the use of tap water (i.E. No remedy is worried) and an electrical cutting-edge-day-day is used to introduce ions into the body thru sweat-glands. The mechanism of treatment of hyperhidrosis via Iontophoresis isn't well understood but is idea to in some manner incorporate the obstruction of the mechanism inflicting sweat to glide from eccrine ducts, therefore decreasing the technology of sweat from the dealt with frame element. This treatment requires regular software as epidermal renewal leads to transport once more of sweat manufacturing after a while.

Due to anatomical and purposeful constraints, Iontophoresis is fine for palmar and plantar hyperhidrosis (excessive sweat in fingers and in toes). Off-late, manufacturers have also provide you with gadgets to deal with other frame elements including face and underarms via Iontophoresis.

Iontophoresis Devices

Iontophoresis is run via specialized clinical devices. The Iontophoresis tool, at its center is certainly an electrical circuit that passes contemporary through the part of body this is located inside the trays entire of tap water, and has 3 fundamental additives:

A supply of electrical modern-day

Trays to immerse the hand/toes into faucet water and

Wires to attach the current-day supply to the tray.

RA Fischer, Drionic, Hidrex and Idromed are a number of the famous manufacturers of Iontophoresis gadgets for hyperhidrosis. These machines are noticeably similar, however may also have enormous variations in terms of the convenience of utilization, manage options, cutting-edge kind, cutting-edge supply type and so forth. The devices variety upwards of $4 hundred with extra expensive ones costing a good buy more. You can also make a primary Iontophoresis device at home (commands).

Below are a few pix of well-known Iontophoresis machines:

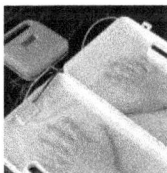

Idrostar

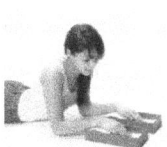

Drionic Hands

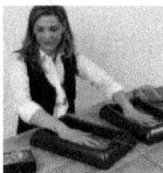

Hidrex

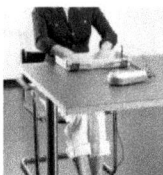

Idromed

Is Iontophoresis Effective?

It isn't totally understood how Iontophoresis treats hyperhidrosis. As a give up end result, you'll get very polar feedback and regularly unsubstantiated claims on internet (the manufacturers of the tool claim that Iontophoresis is "mounted" to be powerful for hyperhidrosis, a few others claim that it does no longer artwork).

However, as with maximum such matters, the reality is someplace in among. There is lots of anecdotal proof that Iontophoresis is robust for hyperhidrosis (which encompass the author), and a large style of patients have claimed to appearance effective, long lasting results for his or her hyperhidrosis situation thru Iontophoresis. Over the course of previous few years of my attempt to understand greater approximately hyperhidrosis and taking to a massive style of sufferers via this net web site, I in my opinion trust that this treatment possibility, if accomplished nicely, works for max of the human beings. Scientific research moreover backs the efficacy of iontophoresis for hyperhidrosis remedy.

Another interest – no critical negative results have been ascribed to the Iontophoresis. So it is able to be truely without a doubt well worth attempting if you have no longer already completed that. There can be little or no to lose and lots to benefit.

How Iontophoresis is completed?

At the maximum fundamental, that is how Iontophoresis works:

1)   Mild electric powered currents are produced the use of a battery or electric powered powered outlet.

2)   The cutting-edge is exceeded down cables to the treatment electrodes which are positioned into trays full of faucet water

3)   Hands and/or toes are then positioned into the trays, finishing the circuit and allowing modern-day to flow into the pores and pores and skin

4)   The affected location is left immersed for about 10-15 minutes

5)   The frequency of treatment is more in the beginning till the signs and symptoms come below manage. Once you have got relief from sweaty hands/toes, the frequency may be diminished to hold the equal (e.G. Once each week)

6)   Treating first rate areas of the body employs the identical method, besides that electrodes are covered with the useful aid of absorbent sponges soaked in tap water and placed onto the remedy vicinity

The remedy can be effects finished at home unaided.

Iontophoresis Side Effects

Iontophoresis is generally taken into consideration safe, and element results are usually restricted to moderate "pins and needles" tingling and slight reddening of pores and skin. In just a few times, painful stinging, itching, small vesicles and mild shocks can also arise. For most people, the initial few instructions are mildly discomforting, however no longer painful. A lot relies upon at the Iontophoresis system being used and the shape of contemporary – pulsed modern-day-day generally outcomes in lots less inflammation compared to direct current. Also, software application of a jelly primarily based definitely product on any

111

exposed reduce/rash on the pores and skin of the vicinity being treated can considerably lessen the soreness.

Who need to no longer do Iontophoresis?

While Iontophoresis has minimal side effect and is in popular suitable for optimum people, you must constantly get a certified medical doctor's recommendation in advance than starting this remedy. Specifically, the subsequent classes of patients want to no longer undergo Iontophoresis:

Pregnant ladies

Patients with cardiac pacemaker

Patients with epilepsy

Patients with most cancers

Patients with swollen, damaged, or inflamed pores and pores and skin at the areas to be treated

Patients with metallic implants within the direction of the modern-day (orthodontic braces are usually taken into consideration stable)

MiraDry

MiraDry, is the trademark name of a non-invasive microwave-based totally generation for the treatment of underarm (axillary) hyperhidrosis. It grow to be advanced via the usage of Miramar Labs in 2006 and had been given FDA clearance 2011. Currently, this way is available high-quality for underarm hyperhidrosis and does not deal with hyperhidrosis for palms or ft

How MiraDry Works

While the technical records are complicated, at the maximum easy diploma MiraDry works via way of directing a pulse of immoderate power microwaves to the sweat glands – producing warmness that destroys the sweat glands in the underarm place, for this reason curing the man or woman of underarm hyperhidrosis.

In parallel, a non-stop cooling device protects the outer layer of the pores and skin even as warm temperature keeps to unfold into the region in which sweat glands are living, ensuing in mobile thermolysis. Sweat glands do no longer regenerate, so once destroyed, the greater sweat glands are anticipated to be honestly disabled.

How MiraDry is used

Outpatient health practitioner visits for MiraDry treatment usually take one hour at some stage in which a scientific medical doctor administers neighborhood anesthesia (usually lidocaine injections

Then he/she makes use of the MiraDry hand held tool to supply electromagnetic power non-invasively to the underarms.

The MiraDry tool cools the outer layer of the pores and pores and skin and sufferers typically enjoy little to no pain all through the system.

There is minimum to no downtime afterwards. Most sufferers are capable of go back to normal sports activities sports or artwork right after the device, and may commonly resume exercise inside severa days.

A slight over the counter ache treatment and ice packs are commonly encouraged for some days

For a few times, it may require up to 2 strategies to without a doubt ruin the sweat glands within the vicinity.

 Side Effects

Common aspect effects of MiraDry consist of

Mild to slight transient swelling and pain inside the remedy vicinity (usually lasting approximately one week)

Mild numbness or altered sensation of the pores and pores and skin within the underarm vicinity (can final severa months)

In unusual instances, it is been said that the procedure may additionally additionally spoil different nerve cells inside the vicinity causing numbness within the hands and palms

Note that his method within reason new, so the full amount of aspect results or long time effectiveness isn't always acknowledged. Good statistics, but, is that compensatory sweating (sweating on one-of-a-kind body components, common after ETS surgical remedy) has no longer been hooked up to be a problem.

MiraDry Cost

The price of the manner depends on the issuer, facilities and the location, however it significantly variety among $1,500 – $4,000 for a single session (you can require up to 2 instructions)

Botox

How Botox works

Botulinum toxin is a protein and is one of the most acutely deadly pollution appeared. Botox is one of the forms of botulinum toxin that is available for numerous splendor and scientific techniques. It is a completely well-known substance used for cosmetic talents (e.G. Wrinkle removal, face lifts and so forth.).

Botox, even as injected into the affected regions can manage hyperhidrosis via using manner of quickly blockading the chemical alerts from the nerves that stimulate the sweat glands. When the sweat glands don't get keep of chemical signals, the excessive sweating stops in the handled region. The distinct areas of the frame are not affected and hold to sweat as earlier than. The effect is brief and lasts about 6 – 8 months after which the remedy is needed over again to hold the results.

How Botox is used

Botox is administered underneath the pores and skin through injections. The medical doctor can also follow the following steps:

Perform Iodine Starch Test: This step identifies the vicinity accountable for hyperhidrosis. Doctor will paint the underarm are with iodine solution. After it dries up, she will lightly sprinkle the area with starch powder. The hyperhidrotic place will boom a deep blue-black shade in about 10 mins

Prepare remedy area: The physician will circle the affected place with a surgical marker, and then smooth area indoors circle with alcohol.

Map area for injection: Using a surgical pen and fashionable ruler, the medical health practitioner will mark injection factors approximately 1.Five to two cm apart.

Inject BOTOX® product: The physician will then count number number the injection elements and allocate recommended dosage of BOTOX answer in step with injection, primarily based on 50 Units consistent with axilla. Then she will be capable of inject to a depth of approximately 2 mm. After injection, smooth handled vicinity with alcohol.

Side consequences

BOTOX® can cause immoderate facet results together with:

dry mouth,

pain or pain on the injection website,

tiredness,

headache,

neck pain,

Eye issues: double vision, blurred imaginative and prescient, reduced eyesight, drooping eyelids, swelling of your eyelids, and dry eyes.

In a few times, the affected person also can get an hypersensitive reaction. This can also itching, rash, purple itchy welts, wheezing, hypersensitive reactions signs, or dizziness or feeling faint.

BOTOX® is accredited by means of the FDA to deal with the signs and signs of excessive underarm sweating whilst drug treatments used at the pores and pores and skin (topical) do no longer art work well sufficient.

Endoscopic thoracic sympathectomy (ETS)

ETS is the most publicized treatment opportunity for Hyperhidrosis (mainly Palmar Hyperhidrosis) on internet, and the nice that earns the maximum cash to the scientific professional community! However, this is the maximum invasive remedy option, and ought to be taken into consideration as a remaining inn due to the reality it may (and regularly does) reasons essential, irreversible detail results which includes compensatory sweating (immoderate sweating on massive regions of the body or at some point of), hypotension, arrhythmia, and heat intolerance.

While internet search can also moreover moreover deliver a exceptional have an effect on, ETS need to not be the number one choice to be taken into consideration for treating hyperhidrosis because of the potentially severe terrible aspect results of the approach.

How Surgery for Hyperhidrosis Work

In easy terms – the ETS gadget blocks the transmission of nerve signals (from sympathetic nerve system) from the spinal column to the sweat glands and to therefore prevent those nerve alerts from "turning on" the sweat glands.

The method is achieved with the affected individual underneath favored anesthesia. A miniature digital digital camera is inserted into the chest under the armpit. The surgeons then lessen or damage the nerve paths related to the overactive sweat glands – this requires collapsing of the lungs on both facets one after the opposite.

Side Effects of Surgery for Hyperhidrosis (ETS)

The most regularly complained drawback of ETS surgical treatment is compensatory sweating – i.E. Sweating more than earlier than in a special part of the frame - this takes region almost all of the time, despite the truth that the degree to which compensatory sweating happens also can moreover range affected individual to affected character. Compensatory sweating is immoderate sweating that takes place at the decrease returned, chest, stomach, legs, face, and/or buttocks because of ETS surgical procedure. It can be in addition or maybe more excessive than the authentic sweating trouble.

Other aspect effects of ETS encompass:

Reduction in coronary heart rate: While for almost all of sufferers this is of no give up end result, patients who have an abnormally low coronary heart fee or problem with their coronary heart's electric powered powered conduction device can be severely affected. Patients which may be exceedingly competitive athletes that could require compensatory increase in coronary coronary heart fee or vascular tone with exercising also are impacted.

Gustatory sweating – Patients who growth this problem phrase prolonged sweating whilst they'll be eating. This occurs in about 1% of patients

Horner's syndrome – When this occurs, the affected character notes 3 findings on the side of the face wherein the stellate ganglion changed into injured. These include a mild drop within the eyelid, a small or slim student, and the dearth of sweating on that component of the face.

Surgery for Hyperhidrosis (ETS) – Key Considerations

The ETS system is generally irreversible, and comes with non-trivial dangers of component outcomes. This want to be considered because of the fact the remaining inn, or maybe then, the functionality blessings want to be weighted cautiously in opposition to the functionality thing impact. There are numerous different extra secure options to be had that may go for maximum of the patients and those have to be evaluated first earlier than considering surgical procedure.

Local Underarm Surgery

How Local Underarm Surgery Works?

Besides ETS mentioned above, there's an change, lots much less risky surgical alternatives for sufferers with underarm hyperhidrosis. The close by surgical operation works with the resource of eliminating/incapacitating the sweat glands in the underarm vicinity so that they can not produce sweat anymore.

The approach requires sweat glands to be localized in a instead small place – making underarm vicinity the proper candidate. The neighborhood surgical remedy isn't always but accomplished for Palmar, Plantar, Facial or Truncal hyperhidrosis because the sweat glands in the ones regions are nicely allocated, making the challenge of getting rid of them masses extra difficult.

There are more than one variations inside the approach the physician can use to disable the sweat gland inside the underarm area – at the side of curettage, excision, liposuction, and laser or a aggregate of them. The technique does now not typically require generalized anesthesia. The quit end result of a a achievement surgical operation is usually a everlasting consolation from excessive sweat from the underarm region.

Side Effects

The sweat gland removal surgical procedure for underarm region is typically safe. However masses depends on the unique technique used for the surgical treatment, and the enjoy of the clinical professional in figuring out the sweat glands and disabling/destroying them efficiently.

It ought to be be conscious that the usage of Laser for destroying sweat glands, at the identical time as promising, is pretty present day and the extended-time period outcome and facet effects of this method aren't properly understood. Also, excision (i.E. Complete elimination of sweat glands) also can bring about severe headaches (e.G. Lack of capability to transport arm) and ought to consequently be averted in desire of diverse strategies.

The vital aspect effect of ETS surgical procedure – i.E. Compensatory sweating is typically now not a issue effect of nearby underarm surgical remedy. Just like different surgical techniques, there can be usually the danger of infection if the pores and skin setting out isn't always well covered. Also, the patients may additionally have brief pain and bruising on the surgical operation website online. The surgical operation moreover consequences in minor scars on the internet web page of the surgical procedure.

Local Underarm Surgery: Considerations

If you are thinking about Local Underarm Surgery for Axillary Hyperhidrosis, ensure that the clinical physician is professional and characteristic added top consequences within the beyond. While the above phase also can have made the surgical operation appear like a clean one (discover sweat glands, break them, completed), it's miles a protracted way from that. Spotting the sweat glands and destroying them is a pretty professional technique and the outcomes are especially variable from health practitioner to medical doctor. If the primary surgical procedure does not provide the supposed discount in sweating, your physician might also additionally endorse a 2nd surgical procedure to take out the remaining sweat glands which have been missed the number one time.

Alternative Treatments

Diet Control

Diet manage treatment works at the number one that certain food can increase the sympathetic nerve sensitivity and if the intake of such meals is ceased, the nerve interest will lessen, because of this lowering the amount of sweat produced.

It isn't scientifically studied or verified, but the decrease in intake of following components has been stated to bring about lower of excessive sweat situation:

1.Alcohol: When you drink a tumbler of alcohol, your blood vessels widen, in step with the University of Wisconsin's Center for Alcohol Studies and Education. Although this can purpose your frame to lose warm temperature in the end, to begin with it may purpose you to sweat.

2.Cigarettes

three.Caffeine: Caffeine is a stimulant that causes your heart to triumph over quicker and increases your metabolic fee. When your metabolic price will boom, your body burns extra strength, which in flip will boom your temperature and makes you sweat. Hot coffee and tea can make you sweat even extra without a doubt due to the fact the temperature of the beverage is warm.

4.Certain tablets

5.Certain elements: Pepper, spices

Herbs

Natural dietary dietary dietary supplements have lengthy been used to help deal with immoderate sweating. These supplements are commonly applied in treating hyperthyroidism, or overactive thyroid -- one of the main reasons of immoderate perspiration. Other beneficial dietary supplements may additionally additionally encompass sage, witch hazel and eucalyptus.

Sage can be one of the maximum usually used natural nutritional dietary supplements in treating immoderate sweating. Sage may be beneficial in treating several situations related to excessive perspiration, which consist of night time time time sweats and menopause-related warmness flashes. Sage is a effective astringent, which means that that that it has the capacity to cause tissue contraction, consisting of contraction of your pores and pores and pores and skin.

Chapter 11: Managing Hyperhidrosis

↵"Attitude is a touch element that makes a big distinction." – Winston Churchill

Truth is: Hyperhidrosis affects existence – every so often severely. While there are various remedy options available to govern it higher, there are specific strategies to govern excessive sweat as well.

Persistence

Most of the treatments of hyperhidrosis are brief in nature. Moreover, for lots of them, it calls for a while earlier than the remedy even begins to make a wonderful (e.G. Iontophoresis, antiperspirants). If I were to select out out one hassle that separates hyperhidrosis sufferers from hyperhidrosis "managers" is staying power.

Prepare a calendar on your iontophoresis remedy (if you use iontophoresis) and preserve on with that. If you're using antiperspirants, make it a ordinary to apply the antiperspirant earlier than you doze off every day. If you take remedy, make sure which you don't pass doses even whilst you start feeling better.

It's very easy to give up the remedy plan if there may be no obvious difference for your situation in some days/weeks. Sometimes, all it takes is that extra push to take it to the next day/week in advance than the treatment starts offevolved to artwork. It's even a great deal much less complicated to turn out to be lax on the remedy plan once it virtually works and immoderate sweat is now not a problem. Avoid the temptation, and you will be a hyperhidrosis "supervisor" for life!

Get Organized

Getting organized is an vital step towards vital a existence this is minimally impacted through hyperhidrosis sweat. Keep your excessive sweat equipment nearby on the same time as you need them – which means that:

Organize Wardrobe – get cotton undergarments (to soak up sweat), and dark colored garments (just so sweat stains aren't seen). Get cotton footwear (e.G. Converse footwear) that permit your feet to breathe and sweat to dry off.

Organize Work Bag - Keep antiperspirants, wipes, sweat pads and masses of others. To your paintings bag. That procedures, you can in no manner be stuck at work with out your hyperhidrosis equipment.

Organize Furniture – If you have a say in it, get timber desks with out glass pinnacle. Glass tops are smooth to smudge specifically in case you be tormented by means of palmar hyperhidrosis

Mobile Phone – get a hold in thoughts prevent apparent cover, and a leather cover to your touchscreen cellular telephone. That strategies, you couldn't purpose ugly sweat smidges on the cellular telephone

Tell Your Loved Ones

A lot of sufferers affected by hyperhidrosis in no way tell everybody approximately it, and that reasons strain. In a number of times, the patients do now not even inform their on the spot own family for the priority of being ridiculed. Take my advice – tell individuals who love you about your scenario. You will enjoy higher, and more cushty with their help. If you want to cowl your hyperhidrosis from your partner/siblings, that is a huge source of pressure thru itself. Chances are – they may not love you any a great deal a good deal less on your hyperhidrosis and will handiest offer words of encouragement.

Get Involved

This one comes from my personal experience. If you have got got suffered with hyperhidrosis, you may gain immensely with the resource of connecting with remarkable sufferers with reminiscences like your self. In this day and age, there are various smooth methods to do this – begin a blog, make a contribution to at least one, take part in boards and a few thing else is simple for you. The aspect is – you in no way understand whose lifestyles you may contact via using sharing your hyperhidrosis revel in. And in case you do, that's a extraordinary feeling that makes living with hyperhidrosis a touch a whole lot much less painful.

Chapter 12: Heavy Sweating: How To Stop Hyperhidrosis

There are a set of ideals approximately the manner to stop hyperhidrosis, alongside element some of trouble. If you're most of the tens of tens of millions who battle with severe underarm sweating, you then understand what I suggest. This located up will check the hassle and list some of the unique remedy options.

Extreme underarm sweating is greater not unusual in comparison to you may think. It may be the stand up from a plethora of reasons. Some of these function our heredity, even as others can be from ingredients we consume or drug remedies we perform. Caffeine and alcohol need to even deliver the disorder on. But, no matter the aspect, there are techniques to prevent too much sweating.

The maximum not unusual alternative is utilizing a selected antiperspirant. I'm no longer talking about air freshener indexed here. There is a huge distinction among each that masses of people do not recognize.

Antiperspirants encompass aluminum salts that deodorants do no longer. Aluminum salt works in enclosing sweat channels that produce perspiration and sweat. It protects in competition to the sweat from developing to the ground of the pores and skin.

Deodorants as a substitute simply paintings to dispose of smells, as a quit end result their call.

There have been hundreds of humans claim that antiperspirants had been the cause for breast maximum cancers, however not something of the sort has ever earlier than been examined.

What antiperspirants need to do is to get worse the pores and pores and skin in a few people. This may want to make your underarms pink and even itchy at times. A lot of air fresheners will in fact no longer create this considering that they do now not comprise the very equal factors.

If you've got problem in finding an antiperspirant in order to absolutely protect in opposition to too much sweating, speak together with your physician concerning trying a more powerful prescribed antiperspirant.

Other techniques in locating out the superb methods to surrender hyperhidrosis feature:

Surgery - I will not move into this area because it isn't always that common these days. It is viable to operatively do away with sweat ducts to treatment too much sweating, but it needs to be a remaining wish.

Botox - This has tested to paintings distinctly properly to prevent excessive sweating. It might also likewise be protected for your fitness plan too. Botox treatments may additionally want to keep away from the nerves from inducing the sweat glands. Keep in mind that at the same time as Botox has determined to be effective it is able to be unsightly, and it exceptional lasts for type of 6-eight months preceding to you will need to duplicate the procedure over again.

Iontophoresis - With this method to lower sweating, the area of the trouble is despatched low degrees of electrical modern-day which then near down the sweat ducts. The treatment could no longer harmed, however tests have clearly verified that it is virtually no superb than simply making use of an antiperspirant.

In locating out how you can stop hyperhidrosis those treatments must offer you with a few an lousy lot wished help. There also are a few exclusive herbal techniques of having rid of the problem that you may find out below. Don't permit this problem retain to manipulate your life. It is treatable.

What You Need to Know

Too a whole lot sweating is a normal trouble, mainly of the hands, underarms and soles. It can be distressing and can have a extreme have an effect on on your life. Sometimes, damaged people steer clear of social call with others due to embarrassment about the trouble. Nonetheless, the sickness is usually treatable.

Chapter 13: Exactly What's Intense Sweating?

Regular sweating assists to keep the body temperature strong in warm weather, inside the path of a fever, or whilst exercising. Too a exquisite deal sweating (hyperhidrosis) indicates that you sweat an extended manner extra in assessment to not unusual. Even while you are not warmness, , or workout, you're making a gaggle of sweat.

Too a great deal sweating is diagnosed into three types (as adheres to). It is important to understand which kind you have got, due to the fact the motives and remedy plans are pretty diverse.

Primary (idiopathic) focal hyperhidrosis

This implies that too much sweating develops in one or more of the complying with focal locations: arms of the palms; soles of the feet; underarms (axillae); face/scalp.

You sweat usually at the the rest of the body. It has the tendency to be in share - that is, every fingers, every feet, each underarms, and so forth., are inspired. The unique purpose is not understood and it isn't always associated with every extraordinary issues. (The phrase idiopathic ways of unidentified supply.) It absolutely seems that the gland in those areas are overactive or extra touchy than common. In some humans, it is able to run inside the family so there may be a few genetic trouble associated with growing it. It generally first establishes underneath the age of 25, but it is able to create at any shape of age. Males and female are in addition inspired. It is not unusual and affects about 3 in 100 human beings.

The severity can also moreover need to range occasionally. It may also moreover moreover come and skip and may be worsened with the useful resource of triggers collectively with pressure and tension, feeling, particularly spiced food, and warmth. Anxiety concerning the sweating itself may moreover moreover make it worse. Nevertheless, for max of the instantaneous, in reality not whatever obvious induces the sweating. It usually be an enduring sickness, but symptoms and signs and symptoms enhance in hundreds of times in time.

If you have got have been given the ordinary signs and signs of maximum critical focal hyperhidrosis, you normally do not need any form of examinations. Your medical doctor may moreover moreover endorse severa methods (under) if widespread antiperspirants do not artwork well.

Secondary focal hyperhidrosis

This is unusual. It indicates that the an excessive amount of sweating happens in a sure focal issue of the body. Yet, in evaluation to fundamental focal hyperhidrosis, there's a regarded or most likely motive. For example, a spinal illness or damage can also bring about sweating in a single leg. Any focal sweating that isn't symmetrical (this is, simply in a unmarried hand, or one leg, and many others.) may furthermore recommend a secondary deliver in preference to primary focal hyperhidrosis which is normally balanced. Your medical health practitioner might also additionally moreover endorse some examinations to in want of a hidden motive if one is suspected.

Generalised hyperhidrosis

This way which you sweat extra than normal sooner or later of. This is an awful lot much less commonplace compared to primary focal hyperhidrosis. Nonetheless, it is commonly triggered through a hidden scientific scenario. A complete collection of issues can bring about a generalised advanced sweating. For instance: tension illnesses, severa coronary heart troubles, damage to nerves in the spinal cord, facet-consequences to specific drug treatments, superb hormonal problems (collectively with an overactive thyroid glandular), infections, unique cancers, and so forth. If you have got surely generalised hyperhidrosis your health practitioner is probable to take a look at you and perform a touch assessments to discover the supply.

Treatment is based totally upon upon the cause.

Essential Information

The majority of human beings produce approximately a litre of sweat every day, however people with hyperhidrosis (concerning 2-3 % of the population), should produce up to ten instances as drastically.

Excessive sweating can be brought on by using the use of illnesses, such as excessive weight, diabetic troubles and high blood pressure. It typically stops as quickly because the underlying sickness is treated.

Yet it is also a sickness in its private proper. When the nerves that manipulate sweating do now not function normally, they create consistent sweating in a unmarried or more regions of the body.

"The fingers, the toes and the underarms (underarm) are the most regular regions," elements out Halford. "The face, the top, the groin, the again and the chest moreover sweat, but now not as normally."

People with immoderate sweating preference they will in truth redecorate the get off. It might not be as clean as that, but there paintings remedies virtually to be had.

Exactly what help is provided?

Changing your way of existence and ordinary tasks can enhance signs and make you experience hundreds greater self-confident.

Self-assist recommendations:

Avoid appeared motives that make your sweating worse, which incorporates rather spiced food or alcohol.

Regularly use antiperspirant spray (in place of antiperspirants).

Avoid tight, restrictive garb and guy-made fibers, along with nylon.

Putting on white or black clothing ought to decrease the symptoms and symptoms of sweating.

Armpit guards might also want to soak up immoderate sweat and defend your clothes.

Use socks that soak up dampness, for instance thick, mild socks fabricated from natural fibers or sports activities socks made to soak up wetness. Avoid synthetics, and exchange your socks at the least two instances a day.

Buy footwears which can be crafted from leather-based-based, canvas or mesh rather than synthetic fabric.

If you are with the resource of an excessive amount of sweating, decide your GP. They may moreover want to indicate the proper medicine. In a few instances you can want to be stated a pores and skin professional (a dermatologist) for added remedy.

Chapter 14: Stopping The Sweat Problem

Although it's one of the matters your frame does that will help you, most human beings would as an alternative go away the sweating to the poolside glass of iced tea. That's due to the fact excessive sweating is a lot like tequila or fact TV-- bearable in small dosages, excruciating at the same time as you're left open to too much of it. This perspiration primer will assist you decide how you can manage, prevent, and accumulate your very very very own perspiring instances.

When your body heats up-- from climate situation, exercise, fear, lingering kisses in your neck-- your mind sends out the message that your device is overheating. The message takes a journey to nerves that reason the more than 2 million sweat glands that lie below your pores and pores and skin. Which's after they ship out wetness through the sweat channels on your pores and skin's floor area. The dissipation out of your pores and pores and pores and skin is what cools down the frame.

"Your hypothalamus gland is a thermostat: If the body's middle temperature will boom, it sends out a message for sweating to start," claims Lawrence Gibson, M.D., a pores and pores and pores and skin professional at the Mayo Clinic. "When the temperature goes down, it shuts the sweat off over again."

Including water, salt, and electrolytes, many sweat may not perfume. What does smell is the aggregate of sweat with numerous other bodily compounds. Your body has shape of sweat glands-- eccrine, which manage frame temperature, and apocrine, which launch scents. The apocrine glands, which may be obtained within the underarms and groin and set up during teenage years, discharge a viscous blend that additionally consists of wholesome proteins and fats. Body smell begins offevolved even as that sweat mixes with bacteria on your pores and pores and skin.

Besides the cooling down characteristic, sweat moreover serves a crucial cause for signaling healthy and everyday bodily feature. "If you're in the middle of an extreme venture and forestall sweating, it's miles a sign of dehydration," Dr. Gibson claims. Sweating offers us a gauge to at the same time as we can be overheating or ought to fill up drinks, he includes, consequently supporting to hold the body's water diploma on course.

Sweating has other blessings. Christine Raffa, proprietor of Raffa Power Yoga in Rhode Island, compares electricity yoga-style sweating to the Native American sweat hotel, which modified into implemented for bodily and religious refinement. Sweating cleanses the pores and skin on the same time as launching contaminants and delivering moisture lower back into the body, she claims.

Although it's miles some thing to sweat whilst you're running, doing yoga, or having intercourse, it's far as an alternative every other to do the entirety over your supervisor' M&M s area. That's why quite a few us utilize a deodorant (to mask odor), an antiperspirant (to gradual the float of sweat), or a mixture of every.

Some ladies, after being attentive to rumors that elements in antiperspirants cause cancer, use various specific strategies similar to the usage of massaging alcohol, blow-drying underarms after showering-- no longer so nutty, for the motive that bacteria is the cause of BO-- or utilizing products crafted from natural substances.

"There's in reality not anything currently informing us [antiperspirant usage] is dangerous," says Marisa Weiss, M.D., oncologist and president of breastcancer.Org. The majority of antiperspirant isn't taken in, she states, and any form of map amount that can be have to actually now not likely make it to the lymph nodes near the underarm. Even if it did, lymphatic drainage flows to the the relaxation of the body, no longer toward the breast, Dr. Weiss says.

Sweat Stop: What to Do

Raffa states she has positioned that the purer the frame obtains-- from enhancing such physical activities as food regimen and workout-- the lots much less she desires to masks smell. "I do no longer really need antiperspirant for every day," she factors out. If you are looking for even extra techniques to downgrade your tropical storm to a moderate drizzle, try the ones exclusive treatments:.

Usage get dressed covers. Place a stick-on dress defend within the underarm of a get dressed or shirt to prevent the warning dark circles (to be had at dressshields.Com).

Watch your weight loss plan. Have a huge assembly showing up? Skip the chook vindaloo the night time time earlier than. Garlic clove, pink onions, and curry all ought to appear via sweat, claims Dee Anna Glaser, M.D., partner trainer of dermatology at Saint Louis University. "We're a hyperclean way of life-- humans take and three showers an afternoon, however although devour rapid food and drinks Diet Cokes," Raffa states, and that has an impact at the heady scent that appears in some unspecified time in the future of a heavy sweating consultation.

Downsize your vices. Carrying introduced weight, smoking, and eating alcohol or caffeine can all enhance sweat as properly, based totally on mayoclinic.Com.

Extreme Sweating: The Signs and Solutions.

If your gland art work greater like a automobile easy than a regularly trickling tap, it can be a signal of a few difficulty greater essential. Diabetes, thyroid troubles, and coronary heart and lung disease all may also need to bring about excessive sweating. Yet it may also be a signal of hyperhidrosis, a prime concerned tool sickness that triggers continual an excessive amount of sweating for no large detail-- commonly within the underarms, fingers, or feet.

Around four million girls address the disease, in keeping with a modern have a look at in Dermatology Journal. (And we do suggest experience. Dr. Glaser recalls one affected man or woman who had a tailor positioned terry fabric wallet in all her pants and skirts so she could possibly dry her arms previous to shaking arms.).

Procedures embody prescription antiperspirants like Drysol, which use immoderate portions of aluminum chloride to save you up gland however moreover can create pores and pores and skin irritability. Surgery has sincerely also been used to brace or reduce the nerves inflicting sweat glands, but the maximum promising treatment is Botox. Understood for plumping out wrinkles, Botox become legal via the usage of the FDA in July for managing underarm hyperhidrosis. "The consequences are superb, and the safety profile is truly accurate-- no huge spread horrible factor consequences," Dr. Glaser claims.

The way takes approximately 10 minutes. Each underarm gets 10 to 20 pics of Botox-- FIFTY milligrams in every pit (topical anesthesia is non-obligatory). People see a large decrease of sweat (even though not a hundred percent) in 2 to a few days, claims Dr. Glaser. Procedures run from $4 hundred to $1,000 in step with underarm and need to be duplicated regarding every 6 to three hundred and sixty five days (even though coverage coverage commonly covers it for hyperhidrosis sufferers).

"I recall a set of people available are suffering with hyperhidrosis and do not understand there can be a remedy that could look after it," says Joel Spitz, M.D., a New York pores and pores and skin professional. "These people are hugging me the subsequent time they see me. They turn out to be being commonplace humans once more."

Chapter 15: Causes

I started to expect that my problem come to be warmth associated. My body temperature modified into usually heat. My breath modified into heat. I come to be stinking badly. What ought to it be? Then I positioned my device. It is nicely known as a manner to take away gallstones however I did now not see virtually everybody speakme approximately it assisting sweating. There are many brilliant motion images explaining the way to do a liver flush similarly to many blog posts discussing the statistics. I determined to do it.

After a 24 hour rapid and downing an olive oil and citrus concoction (which tasted quite proper to me), I changed into walking to the bathroom. Like many others earlier than I successfully flushed loads of gallstones! After the primary week, I observed a lower in the amount of sweat on my underarms. I became coaching and am very lively after I do. I use a ton of strength each day to hold my college students fascinated and engaged within the dialogue. But I wasn't sweating or smelling almost as awful as before. I end up onto some thing. I gave my liver a few weeks relaxation and went in for round 2. Success another time. Within the subsequent week my sweat and the severity of my heady scent end up reduced thru the use of 1/2 of what it modified into earlier than. In reality, I now not sweat in cold weather or air conditioned rooms. I most effective sweat even as my stress is excessive and I am running hard. I no longer want to pin my arms at the same time as I attempt to save throughout the first rate marketplace! This is coming from a person who loves to devour wholesome and junk meals, pizza, hamburgers, workout four – 5 days consistent with week, and sleep handiest 5-7 hours a day! I could frequently eat greasy protein rich materials overdue into the early hours of the morning.

My liver come to be trapping my frame heat it regarded and it have end up displaying throughout my pores and pores and skin. In reality, this is not something new. Chinese medication connects the liver and kidneys to border warmness. Check out the link to look what I imply, very captivating stuff. Http://www.Acupuncture-elements.Org/ultimate-pathogenic-element.Html

During the time I end up building up the warmth in my liver, I advanced a large amount of eye floaters and my hair changed into falling out appreciably more than ever. What in the global is probably taking region!! Well, some years within the beyond my frame started radiating an extraordinary amount of warmth. I become on the identical old American eating regimen. Hey, I'm not complaining right here. I love cheeseburgers and pizza clearly as an entire lot as each person else but some thing become constructing up this warm temperature through the years. On a chilly wet night time I can also need to fog up my component of the auto embarrassingly. You can accept as true with how the tension should collect truly thinking about going out on a date with this little problem.

Another spot I changed into 'trapping warmth' modified into in my palms. My interest as a teacher overseas is pretty stressful at times. A lot is predicted through my clients and I need to present them the entirety I need to provide. Naturally this could reason me to traumatic up in a few unspecified time inside the future of the day. I discovered I typically will be inclined to ball up my arms into tight little fists. By continuously keeping them closed I actually have become expending electricity and contributing to in addition tightening up which ultimately introduced about greater sweating. Look for those little tight spots during your body. Maybe you have got were given them to your face, jaw, hips, shoulders, ft, eyes. Anywhere that isn't always cushty will come again and chunk you.

Chapter 16: Solutions

Maybe your posture is off. Or you have have been given tight hips or psoas. Maybe you have got a lower lower again damage which you by no means took care of this is inflicting one element to tighten up.

Poor posture impacts masses of heaps of human beings round the sector each day. We have end up aware of constantly searching down at our telephones, analyzing at desks searching down at books, sitting in poorly designed chairs, or even reinforcing horrible posture in the fitness center through awful form. Maintaining an brilliant posture all through the day will save you tight spots that cause greater tension and heat to be 'trapped' within the body.

Get into an awesome stretching routine. I imply a honestly proper one. Stretch out your legs, lower back, chest, neck, shoulders, ft, and fingers. This can all be finished in only a few minutes every day.

Make positive your shoulders and top again are cushty too. The yoga roller or a lacrosse ball can help relax your back and shoulders. You do now not want to shop for one but if you discover your shoulders, neck, and decrease returned getting tight too regularly remember making an funding in a easy shiatsu massager just like the only determined right here http://amzn.To/2aHQKKS I to begin with offered the shape of for my spouse because of the fact she always asks me to massage her legs however we determined it too slim and her legs are not even big! But we did positioned this hassle to apply on our shoulders and neck area. I by no means even knew I had tension in my neck. It changed into similar to the ultimate last part of me that I couldn't loosen up myself. They run for about $30 - $forty. They may also even hook as a whole lot because the DC port in your automobile, despite the reality that I don't suggest turning it on while driving! These really help to relieve any tension and get deep into your muscle corporations. They are especially portable and may be used on distinctive elements of your frame like your legs, arms, thighs, or feet. I pretty advise getting one ultimately.

The first step to getting this trapped warmth from your body is through flushing your liver. I swear by means of the usage of the usage of it. Nothing else had ever had any superb impact on me till I did this on a whim. I idea it become cool to be sincere. Flushing gallstones out of one's body almost on command for a more healthy body? I'm thinking about it! The method I used is the one stated through Andreas Moritz. He information this tremendous technique in his e-book available here http://amzn.To/2aJseIW. Many human beings have completed a couple of liver flushes efficiently and successfully. If you're uncertain if this is steady for you or you have got preexisting health situations please seek advice from a health practitioner first. I will not be held liable for harm or death. Ok, now that this is out of the way allow's preserve.

Here is how I did mine:

For approximately four-five days previous to the flush you want to drink normal save sold apple juice. The acid used to make the reasonably-priced juice facilitates to soften the gallstones for a a hit flush. I drank about 3 – four cups an afternoon.

1.In the morning, devour very little. Make certain to now not consume any fats. I actually ate grapefruit. I later drank the rest of my apple juice.

2.At 3pm forestall eating or eating some difficulty.

three.Mix four tablespoons of herbal epsom salts (no delivered perfume) with three cups of water. Put it someplace to kick back otherwise you may gag even as you drink it. This is a laxative you will drink inside the middle of the night.

4.Around 7pm drink 2/three of the laxative your stirred up formerly. Hint: if gag had a taste this will be it. Down that sucker short!

You may also additionally moreover need to run to the relaxation room inside the next half of of of hour so be prepared!

5.Take each exceptional 2/3 of this adorable drink round 9pm and get prepared to camp out round the rest room.

6.Your colon is getting cleansed so most effective the gallstones will come out later. Around 11pm mix ½ cup of more virgin (terrific) olive oil with 1/3 – 2/3 cups of hand squeezed nutrition C juice (grapefruit, lemon, and so on). MAKE SURE THERE IS NO PULP. Mix or shake that up actual properly.

7.Take the juice mixture to your mattress and brush your enamel, exchange your clothes and so on. You will handiest be mendacity down until morning.

8.Down all the juice and oil mixture. Mine tasted pretty particular. Immediately lie down in mattress! Do now not upward thrust up or lay to your factor. Lay flat on your all over again for the subsequent few hours for this to nicely paintings.

nine.You may moreover additionally experience gallstones rolling from your liver at this element this is surely amazing. My first time I felt a hint pressure this is normal, no longer something became caught. Try and nod off. If you can not its adequate neither have to I, I changed into so worried. Stay flat! Listen to a podcast or something.

10.You may additionally additionally find out your self having to go to the bathroom within the night time time. Its good enough, pass in advance. You can also start to see your first signal of stones. They will appear like inexperienced sand or round shaped ovals or maybe summary shapes of yellow green. Go lower returned to bed and hold to go to the toilet inside the morning.

eleven.When you wake take some other 2/3 of that horrible laxative mixture to help flush greater stones out. You do no longer need to move away them in your body. They are ldl ldl cholesterol and that is gross.

12.Take the final of that water made in hell 2 hours later. You need to start to shoot out quite masses water by means of using manner of the after noon. Congratulations! You are completed!

13.Drink a few juice then devour some easy fruit and regularly make your manner once more to normal meals within the direction of the day just to be safe.

The most important a part of getting over your sweating is to widely recognized that it's miles natural. Hear me out. When you sweat you annoying up which reasons extra anxiety. The anxiety produces greater strength expenditure in the shape of heat which motives extra sweat this is further suppressed with the aid of manner of your growing tension. See the vicious cycle?

For the number one few weeks you need to return returned to terms with your self and admit that sweating is ordinary. It will seem and in the end it'll subside even within the maximum updated weather. Allow your self to sweat. If you want to location on most effective white tshirts or those grey coloured ones that don't display sweat an excessive amount of. Do it. Get a few cheap shirts that do not healthy too tight. I changed into sporting some brandname sports sports activities t-shirts which had been all designed to healthful tighter across the higher frame. I rapid switched to 3 looser becoming t-shirts. Cotton works properly however I emerge as though sweating within the ones once I first commenced out. You will probable soak those in sweat however do not worry, it's going to get higher rapid. Keep yourself comfortable mainly spherical your shoulders and arms. Breathe slowly in a few unspecified time within the destiny of the day and accept the sweat. Practice aware respiration and consider the cool air entering your frame and the modern air you exhale to radiate the warmth for you.

Chapter 17: Living Anxiety And Sweat Free

Hyperhydrosis, for almost all of humans, is a faced demon. A physical and a intellectual one. People who sweat are regularly on region, they'll be satisfied but from a frightened machine attitude they'll be a mess. Too many switches are left on and their body is being overtaxed. Do you find out your self juggling masses of thoughts at some level in the day?

Keep your hands and palms loose and snug. Continue your slowed breathing at a few level within the day. Make first-rate you aren't keeping your mouth tightly close to. Focus on one issue at a time in choice to looking for to interest on everything at the same time. If you do no longer bear in mind that you have this hassle do that easy exercise for at some point. Take a memo pad and pen with you and write down every single concept you have got from meals, to plans, to the entirety you consciously take a look at. The remaining one being the maximum essential.

Analyzing takes the most strength, attention and day out of your day. What do I suggest? You are the use of down the toll road, as an instance, and begin to consider the auto to the right inside the the the front of you. You begin looking the car and proper away make judgments approximately their preference of car, the use of style, and lots of others. You word a scratch and offer you with a possible state of affairs of methods it happened. Then the automobile flips on its blinker to trade lanes. Then you pick out them for the way they exchange lanes and pass them to stare them down. Look at that hair. Where are they from? Have I visible them earlier than? These are all thoughts that may be exciting whilst analyzing a singular but this plenty pointless inner speak is sufficient to kindle that fireplace in an effort to get you sweating. It might not reveal itself within the beginning but the effect is properly beneath way so even as you make it to the air-conditioned grocery store you're already stressful.

On top of which you start stressful who's looking at you and whether or not or now not they'll be capable of see you sweat or no longer. Within minutes you have got dark spots under your palms and perhaps your lower again. Oh no! Someone may additionally have seen you sweat by using the use of now perhaps even a few! It's getting warmth in proper proper right here! Now your hands are feeling wet and you're now not able to respire deeply. Surprise! Now you are blanketed in sweat! Better get within the vehicle quick! Once you get home you want to exchange your blouse and its pleasant lunchtime! Why me?!

Let's recap. Here is your look at for drastically lowering and ultimately stopping sweating inside the next few weeks:

Relaxing is a essential step to overcoming your sweating trouble. Always look for little things you do like keeping your breath, bouncing your leg on the equal time as sitting, obsessing over certainly one of a kind little problems which you are managing. I find out myself exhaling lengthy gradual breaths to hold my temperature down. I keep my vocal chords unfastened this way and do now not push my tongue around in my mouth as a high-quality deal. I moreover, stopped sucking in my belly out of years of addiction and targeted on in reality loosing my gut. I turn out to be exercising however highly held my belly fat because of the truth I was eating too much. Even in case you are a body builder you do now not need almost as masses food intake as advertising and marketing and advertising and marketing professionals might have you ever don't forget. But this is every other story.

Chapter 18: Hyperhidrosis

Abnormally improved sweating, in greater of that required for law of frame temperature, is known as hyperhidrosis. Underarms, hands and soles are additives of the frame which may be typically affected with this condition. First signs and symptoms and signs and symptoms of hyperhidrosis start typically in childhood or at some point of the teenage years and irregular sweating can keep at some degree inside the entire life.

Usually Hyperhidrosis rise up in parents which is probably healthful. Heat and feelings may moreover prompt hyperhidrosis. Although neurological, endocrine, infectious, and special systemic illnesses can once in a while reason this condition.

Sweating cool the frame. When body temperature is going up, worried system activates sweat glands In hyperhidrosis the nerves liable for this end up an excessive amount of active and ship alerts for more perspiration despite the fact that it is not desired. Excessive sweating will become larger while character is in a demanding situation.

When there may be no specific reason for this case, it is known as primary hyperhidrosis. But unusual sweating can be because of various scientific conditions like diabetes, menopause, low blood sugar, coronary coronary coronary heart attack, and so forth.

In this example the condition is called secondary hyperhidrosis.

Primary heyperhidrosis impacts hands, soles and face. Secondary affects the entire body.

Emotionally triggered hyperhidrosis, localized hyperhidrosis, and generalized hyperhidrosis are 3 wonderful kinds of this situation. No be counted number wide range which for of hyperhidrosis is present all of them purpose emotional issues and stop them sufferers of their each day functioning.

Conventional treatment

Sometimes the everyday antiperspirants don't assist so it's far crucial to benefit out for more potent one. Aluminum chloride hexahydrate is the maximum inexperienced. This must be implemented in the nighttime 2-3 times in step with week to dry pores and skin on armpits, soles or fingers.

On of the choice is Botox injections below the armpit, which prevents the nerves from sending signals that stimulate sweat glands. This is not a everlasting answer because impact lasts for up to six months. To keep the effects this form of remedy need to be repeated.

As a treatment for this form of troubles Iontophoresis is widely identified all through final 50 years. It is unknown the way it works however it is assumed that it in all likelihood rapid blocks the sweat duct.

The manner makes use of water to conduct an electric powered powered present day to the pores and pores and skin a pair times at some stage in the week, for approximately

10-20 mins in line with consultation, accompanied with the resource of a safety software program of treatments at 1- to 3-week durations, depending on the affected individual's reaction. This remedy is painless.

Lasers and surgical operation can assist with hyperhidrosis. Lasers can find out and wreck the underarm sweat glands.

And there's a surgery called thoracic sympathectomy that can be considered as a last motel.

It is s surgical interruption of the sympathetic nerves responsible for sweating. During this operation a part of the nerve deliver to the sweat glands is destroyed.

Sympathectomy is effective but additionally this operation consists of a big danger. Complications can encompass excessive sweating in exceptional components of the body.

Chapter 19: Natural Treatment

Baking soda, lemon and all forms of herbs will help with hyperhidrosis. You can prepare teas, baths and different combinations in your own home.

Apple cider vinegar

Apple cider vinegar acts as a herbal deodorant as it destroys micro organism. It is sufficient to apply vinegar simply one time an afternoon.

Dry cotton pad soak with combination of apple cider vinegar and water (2: 1) and wipe the ground of the body which can be sweating an excessive amount of. Do this each night time time in advance than mattress.

Baking soda

You should purchase a small package deal deal of baking soda in any preserve for a few cents. Therefore, baking soda can be very practical answer in competition to perspiration and unpleasant fragrance of sweat.

Add a pinch of baking soda in a hint water. Rub the skin, allow it dry, and dry with paper towel. At the give up dispose of the rest of the powder.

Black tea

The black tea is rich with tannin, which includes acid that acts as a herbal antiperspirant and effect the glands and reduces immoderate sweating. Boil half of of a cup of water and dip in small bundle of black tea.

Remove tea bags after a minute and positioned them aside on a plate to relax. Put the luggage at the vicinity of the body in which sweating is progressed, depart on for 5 minutes and eliminate them.

Chapter 20: Lemon

Lemon is utilized in opposition to excessive sweating and to govern frame heady scent. Citric acid kills bacteria and acts as a herbal deodorant. It is essential to comprehend that after treatment of the pores and pores and skin with lemon person should keep away from solar.

Cut the lemon in 1/2 of and rub it on underarms. Leave on for 15-half of-hour and then wash skin with cold water.

Antiperspirant tea

For this tea you need 25 grams of sage leaves, 50 grams of horsetail and 25 grams of green walnut shells

Chop sage and horsetail and finely cut up the shell walnuts. Mix with four dL of hot water over. Cover the bowl and depart for 6 hours.

Sage bathtub

To prepare this bathtub you need 50 grams of sage leaf and 3 dL of water. Chop sage leaves and pour warmth water. Cover and go away for 10 mins. Strain the fluid and use the water to easy fingers, soles underarms.

Prevention

Wearing comfortable garments manufactured from herbal materials like wool, cotton, linen or silk will help. These fabric because opposite from synthetics and polyesters have the electricity of absorption and they don't prevent evaporation. During the summer season it's miles advocated to region on a miles broader clothes so the air can freely flow into the frame. The same is going for socks.

He need to be of cotton or wool and exchange them on a every day foundation. Shoes with leather soles might be the first-class preference. Taking care of hygiene i mainly essential. All varieties of merchandise can assist but cleaning soap, powder and antiperspirant are most important. While everyday deodorants handiest masks the fragrance, antiperspirants include energetic materials that block the sweat glands.

Certain diets can also reason immoderate sweating and smell. For start decreasing consumption of caffeine, alcohol and heat, relatively spiced meals will help. Bananas, oranges and tomatoes and eating water will make up for fluid and electrolytes which can be out of area through sweating.

Chapter 21: Symptoms

Hyperhidrosis is characterised through excessive sweating due to the fact the primary symptom.This goes beyond the sweating due to exercising, being in a heat surroundings, or experiencing anxiety or stress.At least one waking episode of the form of hyperhidrosis that typically impacts the face, palms, toes, or underarms takes vicinity each week.Additionally, the bulk of the time, the body sweats on every factors.

When to go to the health practitioner Sometimes, immoderate sweating is an indication of a few problem excessive.

If you experience excessive sweating, dizziness, ache within the chest, throat, jaw, palms, shoulders, or throat, as well as cold pores and skin and a short pulse, you ought to are seeking out clinical interest proper away.

If you revel in any of the subsequent:

Your every day routine is disrupted with the useful resource of sweating; sweating motives emotional distress or social withdrawal; you unexpectedly begin sweating greater than regular; you have were given night time time sweats for no apparent reason.

Causes

Sweating is the frame's manner of cooling itself.When your body temperature rises, the involved device mechanically activates the sweat glands.When you're worried, sweating additionally takes vicinity, especially to your palms.

Defective nerve signals that cause eccrine sweat glands to end up overactive are the inspiration purpose of number one hyperhidrosis.Most of the time, it impacts the arms, soles, underarms, and face.

This sort of hyperhidrosis has no recounted medical purpose.It can be genetic.

An underlying scientific situation or taking top notch medications, like painkillers, antidepressants, and some diabetes and hormonal medicinal capsules, can reason secondary hyperhidrosis.Sweating can also arise inside the path of the frame due to this type of hyperhidrosis.

Some of the topics that would purpose it are:

Troubles with the thyroid, diabetes, menopause, some kinds of maximum cancers, issues of the anxious device, and infections

Complications

Hyperhidrosis-associated complications include:

Infections

Infections of the pores and pores and skin are more commonplace in folks who sweat plenty.

Emotional and social consequences

It may be embarrassing to place on sweat-soaked garments and hands which might be clammy or dripping.Your situation might make it greater tough in order to acquire your artwork and educational dreams.

Diagnosis

The first step in diagnosing hyperhidrosis might be in your clinical clinical physician to inquire about your signs and symptoms and signs and symptoms and clinical information.You may moreover need to have a physical exam or take a few checks to discover what is inflicting your signs and signs and signs and signs.

Tests within the lab

Your physician might also moreover want to test your blood, urine, or extraordinary samples in the lab to appearance if your sweating is due to each unique scientific situation, like hypoglycemia or an overactive thyroid (hyperthyroidism).

Sweat exams

Thermoregulatory sweat check

Sweat take a look at Open pop-up conversation area

Or you could need a check that pinpoints the regions of sweating and evaluates how immoderate your situation is. Two such exams are an iodine-starch test and a sweat take a look at.

www.ingramcontent.com/pod-product-compliance
Lightning Source LLC
Chambersburg PA
CBHW051726020426
42333CB00014B/1178